600 MCQs in Anaesthesia: Clinical Practice

For Churchill Livingstone

Commissioning Editor Timothy Horne
Copy Editor Sukie Hunter
Project Controllers Kay Hunston, Debra Barrie
Design Direction Erik Bigland
Sales Promotion Duncan Jones

600 MCQs in Anaesthesia: Clinical Practice

Neville W. Goodman
MA DPhil FRCA

Consultant Senior Lecturer in Anaesthesia, University of Bristol and Southmead Hospital, Bristol, UK

Chris Johnson
MA MD FRCA

Consultant Anaesthetist, Southmead Hospital and Clinical Lecturer, University of Bristol, UK

SECOND EDITION

Churchill Livingstone
EDINBURGH HONG KONG LONDON MADRID MELBOURNE NEW YORK AND TOKYO 1996

CHURCHILL LIVINGSTONE
Medical Division of Pearson Professional Limited

Distributed in the United States of America by Churchill
Livingstone Inc., 650 Avenue of the Americas, New York, N.Y.
10011, and by associated companies, branches and
representatives throughout the world.

First edition 1987
Second edition 1996

ISBN 0 443 048355

British Library Cataloguing in Publication Data
A catalogue record for this book is available from the British
Library.

Library of Congress Cataloging in Publication Data
A catalog record for this book is available from the Library
of Congress.

The
publisher's
policy is to use
**paper manufactured
from sustainable forests**

Produced by Longman Singapore Publishers (Pte) Ltd
Printed in Singapore

Contents

Preface

This is the second edition of a book that provides examination practice at Multiple Choice Questions on Clinical Practice for the Fellowship of the Royal College of Anaesthetists (FRCA). The questions are arranged in mock papers of 30 MCQs, to allow candidates to time themselves answering questions similar to those they will encounter in the actual examination, and each paper is followed by annotated answers. The book will help with the need to get a feel for MCQ papers before being faced with the real thing in the examination hall.

Although many of the simpler topics are relevant to the Primary FRCA, the examination that replaced the Part One examination, the book is mainly suited to providing revision for the second part of the FRCA, the examination that replaced the Part Three examination. Candidates for the European Diploma of Anaesthesiology should also benefit.

Unlike those books of MCQs arranged under topic headings, candidates will have to be adaptable, not only to the topic changing from question to question, but also to the degree of difficulty – and, as is bound to happen in the actual examination, candidates will find some questions that they cannot answer.

There are few questions in this second edition that are exactly the same as in the first edition. About one-fifth of the questions are entirely new, or have had at least three of the branches altered. Many of the others have had one or two branches replaced, and most have had the wording altered to make the questions clearer. The answers to many questions have been expanded.

Many of the changes reflect changes in knowledge and in anaesthetic practice since the first edition. Some alterations for this second edition came after trainee anaesthetists in Bristol pointed out errors in the first edition and we thank them. We are not afraid to receive similar comments about this edition, but remind candidates that in the actual examination they will never know what the examiners' answers are. If this book allows candidates to identify gaps in their knowledge before the examination, or if it encourages discussion between candidates and tutors about what is a correct answer, then it will have served its purpose.

Bristol, 1996

N.G.
C.J.

Introduction to the second edition

Since the first edition, the three-part examination structure has become established. The examination is about to revert to a new two-part structure. The new structure gives this new edition a better focus, because the first edition was always better geared to testing knowledge for the old Part Three, and this edition can now be aimed properly at the new Final FRCA examination.

We have modified the structure of the first edition, in which 10 'papers' of 60 mixed questions were to be each answered in sittings of $1\frac{3}{4}$ hours. Recognising that $1\frac{3}{4}$ hours is a long time to put aside for undisturbed study, there are now 20 'papers' of 30 mixed questions, each paper to be answered in 45 minutes.

Progress in clinical anaesthesia means that some 'true' answers in the first edition are now 'false'. Some drugs have become obsolete, some to be replaced by new ones. Anatomy changes little, but even some of those questions have been altered.

There are few questions that are precisely as they were in the first edition. MCQs are better if stem and branches are always complete sentences, so we have altered those that were not. We have simplified many questions and, we think, made them easier. Practice questions should not be easier than those in the examination, but candidates did say after the first edition that some were perhaps too testing – and too discouraging. Many answers are now given more fully. Readers are invited to write to the authors if they find an incorrect answer, though we have tried to check them all. But bear in mind that of greatest importance is your overall score on a paper; and that in the examination hall you will never know what the examiners think is the correct answer.

Introduction

There are two things that you must do to pass the examinations for the Fellowship of the Royal College of Anaesthetists (FRCA): you must reach a certain level of knowledge; and you must know how to present it to the examiners. This is the second of two books that are more concerned with the second of these requirements; they will also help you to assess your level of knowledge, but they should not be treated as sources of knowledge.

In the first book of 600 MCQs we set questions on physiology, pharmacology and clinical measurement. This book covers a full range of clinical topics on which you may be questioned in both the written and oral sections of the Final examination: these include medicine, surgery, applied pharmacology, anatomy, and both general and specialised questions on anaesthesia and intensive care.

The standard textbooks are the best source books of basic knowledge for the FRCA. The more specialised texts, reviews in the journals, and discussion with others should be used to build upon this knowledge – to update it and to find faults in it. You cannot expect to pass an examination unless you work for it: the more clinically oriented the examination, the more importance you must place on gaining wide experience in clinical anaesthesia. You must avoid the danger of working too much 'at the books'.

Many people think that the key to these exams is to go on a course, and there is no doubt that courses can be extremely useful. They should, however, be thought of as a means of aiming one's studies in the right directions; it is disappointing to find that many people will attend a course 2–3 months before the hurdle of a major examination apparently without having done any work. This is foolhardy. To get the most out of a course, you should have covered some of the groundwork beforehand. Once you have acquired what you hope to be sufficient knowledge, then is the time that these books should be of help to you.

HOW TO ANSWER MULTIPLE CHOICE QUESTIONS

The format of the MCQs in the FRCA examination is a stem and five branches. The stem may be short ('Mitral stenosis causes:'), or may be a few lines, for example when presenting a clinical problem. Each of the five branches that follow may be true or false. You score one mark for each correct answer, minus one for each incorrect answer, and, extremely important to the examination technique, you score nothing if you choose not to answer a particular branch. Your actual answers are marked by computer, and so you must eventually put your answers on to special cards that are supplied separately. These cards have the question numbers printed on them and you indicate your answer by filling in a 'true', 'false' or 'don't know' box in pencil.

There are no short cuts or easy ways to answer MCQs. In summary, the best advice is *read the question, don't run out of time and don't guess*. You should answer everything you know, everything you think you know and everything you can work out. Leave any question that is just a guess: if you don't know – leave that branch blank. Only you can know when an 'informed guess' becomes just a guess, and practising MCQs will help.

You must read each stem very carefully: watch out for qualifying words such as 'commonly', 'rarely', 'always' and the like because they can turn what would otherwise be a 'false' into a 'true' and vice versa. Re-read the stem with each statement: it is all too easy to forget the emphasis and exact wording of the stem as you work down the five branches. Watch out for negatives: in the heat of the moment you may fail to see 'not' in a branch. 'May' is an awkward word; one can argue that anything 'may' cause anything else. Try to give the answer relevant to clinical practice: for instance, it is 'true' that atropine may cause bradycardia, but not that propranolol may relieve bronchospasm.

There are some subjects on which questions tend to be particularly confusing: the oxyhaemoglobin dissociation curve is one, the ionic dissociation of drugs is another. These are both subjects in which the wording of stem and branch are crucial. If an option states, 'The saturated vapour pressure of halothane is 243 mmHg', then the answer is clear (if you happen to know!); but the concept and consequences of 'The oxyhaemoglobin dissociation curve is shifted to the left by hypercapnia' can be expressed in a number of different ways – and even then the wording of the stem may alter the answer. When we think that a question is of this type we make a comment about it which you can read along with the answer: we try to point out how a question is confusing.

It is impossible to write an MCQ paper without some of them being ambiguous – or seeming ambiguous to some people. Some of our questions may be ambiguous and we apologise for this, but some of the questions in the actual examination paper will be ambiguous, or will seem so to you in the examination hall, and you must learn how to deal with them.

It is often more difficult to think of false branches than true branches when compiling MCQs. Questions tend to fall into two basic types: the straightforward factual type and the deductive type. Many simple medical questions present facts: a disease and five symptoms and signs that may or may not be features of that disease. A false branch must appear to some candidates to be true or else the question will not discriminate between the good and the poor candidate. The false branches are likely to be: the exact opposite of the true answer (for example, hyperkalaemia for hypokalaemia); an association with a similar disease; or a complete red herring. These last can be very difficult to answer, and you may not be able to find the correct answer in the literature because the connection does not exist. False answers in the deductive type of question include these types, although they may not be so obvious, but also include answers of false logic.

Clinical questions in MCQ examinations often give a short clinical scenario in which the stem is a truncated history with perhaps the results of a few investigations. The branches may ask, for instance, for 'possible' or 'likely' diagnoses. The papers in this book include some questions of this type, but there is no substitute for clinical experience, and that is the best way of improving your performance on applied clinical questions.

A STRATEGY FOR A MULTIPLE CHOICE PAPER

You should have a general strategy for answering an MCQ paper. For those who haven't, we suggest one here. We are not saying it is the only one, but we think it allows efficient use of the time spent answering the paper.

First, read through the questions from the first to the last, answering quickly those of which you are certain of the answers. Mark the branches T or F on the question paper instead of marking the computer card as you go; it will be easier to check your answers. Put a question mark by any stem or branch that you need to think about, or by any answer about which you are uncertain. Put a cross by any stem or branch that you think you will probably not be able to answer at all. It is very important not to dwell on doubtful questions on the first read-through or you may find yourself short of time before you have answered all the questions that you *do* know.

On the second read-through, tackle those that you marked with a question mark; don't be afraid to scribble formulas or graphs on scrap paper to help you with confusing questions. After this second read-through it is worth going back and rechecking the answers – but don't dwell on those that you answered easily on the first read-through or you will find yourself doubting even your most cast-iron certainties. At this stage, transfer the answers that you have made so far to the computer cards and *make sure that you mark the cards correctly*; it is easy to get out of phase between the question numbers and answer numbers. You should now regard these answers as immutable: don't look at the questions again and get on with answering those that you marked with a cross. Answers to these questions you can transfer to the computer cards right away because you will have had plenty of time to think around the subject.

When you have answered all you can, check that you have written your name everywhere that you should have done, and it may be better to leave the examination hall. With essay questions, you should always be able to add more to your answers and you should stay for every precious minute; staying and staring at MCQ answers induces neurosis.

THE MCQ PAPERS IN THIS BOOK

The 600 questions are arranged in 20 'papers' of 30 questions, each paper being a mix of medicine, surgery, applied pharmacology and clinical anaesthesia. We suggest that the best way to test yourself is to try a whole 'paper' *under examination conditions, unseen, in 45 minutes*. The actual examination allows 2 minutes per question, but this includes the time to mark the answer cards. If you take longer than 45 minutes for each 30-question paper you may run out of time in the examination when transferring your answers. The index at the back of the book allows you to find questions under broad subject headings so that you could, if you wanted, answer a number of questions from different papers on, say, cardiology. You will, however, gain nothing if you look at the answers without trying the questions; and there is little to gain from trying a question if you have not done the work on the subject. There are more questions on some topics than on others. Some of the questions in the later papers on these topics are similar to the questions in earlier papers and will allow you to assess whether your factual recall or your understanding of the topic has improved.

HOW TO SCORE YOURSELF

For each branch, score +1 if you marked correctly true or false, or −1 if you marked incorrectly true or false. Score nil for any branch for which you gave no answer. The maximum for each question is thus +5, and the minimum is −5.

Your overall score on a 'paper' will give some idea of your general level of knowledge. We cannot say what score corresponds to a 'pass' in the MCQ in the actual examination but, from our experience of setting mock papers to candidates in the past, you should be looking for 50% at the very least (75/150) for one 'paper', and 70% (105/150) is a very good score.

As well as your overall score it is worth calculating your 'efficiency ratio', which is your number of correct answers expressed as a percentage of your total number of attempted answers. Thus you can get an overall score of 50% by answering 75 branches correctly (an efficiency of 100%) or by answering 85 but getting 10 of them wrong: $85 \times (+1)$ minus $10 \times (−1)$. A low total score with a high efficiency implies that you are certain of what you know but your overall level of knowledge is not enough; a low efficiency ratio means that your knowledge is faulty, or that you are guessing.

Often, candidates going up for the examination ask how many branches they should aim to answer. The only sensible answer to this is that you should answer all that you can. There is no safe number. Certainly, answering only 40% is unlikely to be enough to pass, but merely ploughing on and guessing to bring your total answered up above 50% is unlikely to increase your score because half of your additional answers, if they are just guesses, will be incorrect. Similarly, if you have answered 60%, don't assume that there is no need to answer any more – you may have answered more incorrectly than you think.

Your overall score will indicate your knowledge; your efficiency ratio will point out gross faults in technique of answering; you should also look very carefully at those individual questions at which you scored badly. Using the same reasoning as for the complete paper, you will need to score 3 out of 5 to 'pass' a single question. Think carefully why you did poorly on a particular question. The usual reason is simply lack of knowledge and occasionally you will find a complete gap: an inability to answer any of the branches of a question. A very high negative score (–4 or –5) usually means a lack of understanding of the question rather than lack of knowledge, or a misunderstanding or misreading of the wording. These high negative scores have a great effect on your overall score and perhaps one of the main lessons of this book is to help you to avoid them. As we have stressed before, it is essential to *read each question very carefully*: don't rush at the questions.

THE ANSWERS AND COMMENTS

In the answer section for each paper we give explanations of the correct answers and also make comments, if appropriate, on the form and wording of the question. It is very easy to become side-tracked and obsessed when you get a particular branch wrong which you feel you marked correctly. You may find a book or review which shows you are indeed correct. However, nobody fails the MCQ paper because of one branch that, according to the 'correct' answer, they answered incorrectly: concentrate instead on those questions on which you did badly overall. If you scored –3 on a question about acid–base balance it would be more valuable to go and read a good account of acid–base balance, and to seek help from others, than to feel aggrieved that you think we are wrong on one particular point and waste time laboriously checking each particular branch.

We cannot give full explanations for all the branches in all the questions: that would mean writing a large textbook. Some questions demand more explanation than others and some questions have very short comments. For many of the more important topics we advise you to consult the textbooks if you do badly. There are no references quoted, but it should be possible to answer all the questions in the book from reading of the standard texts.

THE LAST WORD

The examiners try to set clear and unambiguous questions on sensible, mainstream subjects. They are not trying to be devious and trick you into giving incorrect answers. It is often said that MCQs are unfair because they penalise candidates who have read widely, who can always find a reason why 'true' is actually 'sometimes true' or 'maybe true'. But MCQs, unlike the real world of medicine, have to have yes-or-no answers. When testing basic knowledge or general principles of clinical anaesthesia, what the examiner wants to know is whether the candidate can see the wood for the trees.

Paper I Questions

I.1 **Kyphoscoliosis commonly presents the following problems to the anaesthetist:**
  A reduced vital capacity
  B difficult intubation
  C abnormal ventilation/perfusion ratio
  D right heart failure
  E hypocapnia secondary to chronic hypoxia.

I.2 **Clinical features of APUD cell disorders that are important to anaesthetic practice include:**
  A hypocalcaemia
  B high glucocorticoid concentrations
  C ketoacidosis
  D anaemia
  E depression of autonomic activity.

I.3 **Retrobulbar block:**
  A is safer than peribulbar block
  B causes miosis
  C reduces intraocular pressure
  D prevents lacrimation
  E increases the likelihood of vitreous prolapse.

I.4 **Inherited disorders likely to cause problems during anaesthesia include:**
  A malignant hyperpyrexia
  B Huntington's chorea
  C Pierre Robin syndrome
  D Down's syndrome
  E acromegaly.

I.5 **Salicylate overdosage can cause:**
  A coma
  B acidosis
  C haemolysis
  D hypoprothrombinaemia
  E hypofibrinogenaemia.

1

I.6   The use of epidural anaesthesia for retropubic prostatectomy:
A   prevents adequate assessment of blood loss
B   is contraindicated in patients over 65 years of age
C   seldom causes hypotension
D   is contraindicated if the patient is taking aspirin for transient ischaemic attacks
E   is contraindicated in hypertensive patients.

I.7   Appropriate treatment for grand mal seizures occurring after surgical removal of a cortical meningioma includes:
A   intravenous phenytoin
B   thiopentone infusion
C   intravenous mannitol
D   intravenous clonazepam
E   hyperventilation.

I.8   The following are likely after amniotic fluid embolus:
A   cyanosis
B   hypofibrinogenaemia
C   hypertension
D   elevated central venous pressure
E   chest pain.

I.9   A 5-week-old baby boy of 4.1 kg presents with projectile vomiting and is booked for a pyloromyotomy (Ramstedt's procedure). The following are true:
A   he is likely to be hypokalaemic
B   he is likely to be acidotic
C   the need for surgery is urgent
D   atropine 0.015 mg/kg is a reasonable premedication
E   the endotracheal tube must be placed using suxamethonium and cricoid pressure.

I.10 Ketamine:
A is a potent analgesic
B does not depress the cardiovascular system
C is rapidly metabolised in the liver
D prevents aspiration by maintaining laryngeal reflexes
E should not be used in diabetics.

I.11 Drugs likely to cause clinically important release of histamine include:
A propofol
B suxamethonium
C pancuronium
D fentanyl
E d-tubocurarine.

I.12 Suitable anaesthetic techniques for fibreoptic bronchoscopy include:
A spontaneous ventilation with nitrous oxide, oxygen and enflurane
B apnoeic insufflation of oxygen and isoflurane
C local anaesthesia
D air entrainment using a Sanders injector
E IPPV with endotracheal tube, relaxant and opioid.

I.13 The following are true of block of the brachial plexus by the interscalene approach at C6:
A there is no risk of pneumothorax
B there is a risk of injecting into the vertebral artery
C the sheath lies between the anterior and middle scalene muscles
D there will be good relaxation of the shoulder
E there will be a unilateral Horner's syndrome.

I.14 The following are approximate equivalent levels for spinal segment and vertebral body:
A C8 and C7
B T6 and T4
C T12 and T9
D L5 and T12
E Sacral and L1.

I.15 The jugular foramen transmits:
A the inferior petrosal sinus
B the vagus nerve
C the hypoglossal nerve
D the spinal accessory nerve
E the internal jugular vein.

I.16   Acute hypokalaemia:
A   occurs in untreated hyperosmolar non-ketotic diabetic coma
B   precipitates digoxin toxicity
C   occurs when blood flow is re-established to a transplanted kidney
D   occurs during treatment of hyperglycaemia with glucose and insulin
E   follows therapy with a carbonic anhydrase inhibitor.

I.17   The electrocardiographic changes of intraoperative hyperkalaemia include:
A   ventricular fibrillation
B   high peaked T waves
C   U waves
D   ST segment depression
E   ventricular extrasystoles.

I.18   Elevation of jugular venous pressure is associated with:
A   a Valsalva manoeuvre
B   tricuspid stenosis
C   sinus tachycardia
D   constrictive pericarditis
E   tricuspid incompetence.

I.19   Paroxysmal nocturnal dyspnoea is a symptom of:
A   left ventricular failure
B   bronchiectasis
C   pulmonary stenosis
D   ventricular septal defect
E   aortic stenosis.

I.20   The following are found in hypoglycaemic coma:
A   moist tongue
B   low blood pressure
C   reduced tendon reflexes
D   hyperventilation
E   polyuria.

I.21   The following cause generalised pruritus with a rash:
A   mycosis fungoides
B   Hodgkin's disease
C   obstructive jaundice
D   pityriasis rosea
E   shingles (herpes zoster).

I.22 Constipation resulting from reduced gastrointestinal motility is associated with:
   A hyperkalaemia
   B hypothyroidism
   C hypocalcaemia
   D ganglion-blocking drugs
   E parenteral opioid therapy.

I.23 In a patient with dystrophia myotonica:
   A spinal anaesthesia produces muscular relaxation
   B depolarising neuromuscular blocking drugs exert their normal effect
   C non-depolarising neuromuscular blocking drugs do not abolish myotonia
   D non-depolarising neuromuscular blocking drugs produce an enhanced effect
   E diaphragmatic function is not affected by the disorder.

I.24 Histamine H_2-receptor antagonists are of benefit in the treatment of:
   A uncomplicated duodenal ulcer
   B Zollinger–Ellison syndrome
   C Mendelson's syndrome
   D uncomplicated gastric ulcer
   E reflux oesophagitis.

I.25 The following are true of chronic pyelonephritis:
   A frequency and dysuria are the commonest presenting symptoms
   B there is massive proteinuria
   C pyrexia is rare
   D it is the commonest cause of death due to renal failure
   E it is a contraindication to renal transplantation.

I.26 Severe right-sided tracheal deviation is caused by:
   A right-sided pneumothorax
   B nodular goitre
   C collapse of the left lung
   D left-sided empyema
   E left pneumonectomy.

I.27 Classically the pain of:
   A a gastric ulcer is well localised
   B hiatus hernia is well localised
   C cholecystitis radiates to the precordium
   D carcinoma of the stomach is worse after food
   E renal colic radiates around the flank.

I.28   **10 days after a routine emergency appendicectomy a 19-year-old girl is unwell with a swinging pyrexia. The following are true:**
   A   an intravenous pyelogram should be ordered to exclude pyelonephritis
   B   subphrenic abscess is a likely diagnosis
   C   a pleural effusion suggests a postoperative chest infection
   D   she should have an urgent laparotomy
   E   a high urinary white cell count does not necessarily indicate infection of the urinary tract.

I.29   **The following are true of chronic peptic ulceration:**
   A   it probably occurs in one in 10 middle-aged men
   B   a chronic duodenal ulcer never becomes malignant
   C   chronic gastric ulcers commonly become malignant
   D   most patients will eventually need surgery
   E   prepyloric ulcers must be biopsied.

I.30   **Common causes of haematuria include:**
   A   cystitis
   B   hypernephroma
   C   benign prostatic hypertrophy
   D   tuberculosis
   E   glomerulonephritis.

Paper I Answers

I.1 **TFTTF**
> **B** The airway may be difficult but it is not a *common* association.
>
> **E** *Hyper*capnia secondary to hypoventilation may influence management.

I.2 **TTTFF**
> Be careful to note 'important to *anaesthetic* practice'. APUD is Amine Precursor Uptake and Decarboxylation.
>
> **D** Anaemia is not a feature of APUD cell tumours, although any tumour can bleed.
>
> **E** They are if anything associated with sympathetic overactivity.

I.3 **FFTFF**
> **A** The peribulbar route is less likely to produce retro-ocular haemorrhage and there is no risk of inadvertent subarachnoid injection of local anaesthetic.
>
> **B** Retrobulbar block causes pupillary dilation (mydriasis).
>
> **D** The lacrimal gland is supplied from the Vth cranial nerve by fibres originating in the VIIth.
>
> **E** Vitreous prolapse is less likely because retrobulbar block reduces intraocular pressure: to a certain extent **C** and **E** are mutually exclusive.

I.4 **TTTTF**
> **B** Huntington's chorea, now more commonly called just Huntington's disease, is an autosomal dominant. Sensitivity to barbiturates and suxamethonium has been reported.
>
> **E** Although likely to cause problems during anaesthesia, acromegaly is not inherited.

I.5 **TTFTF**
> **C,E** Salicylate overdose is not a cause of haemolysis or hypofibrinogenaemia.

I.6 FFFFF

A Regional analgesia may alter blood loss, but does not prevent assessment.

B Epidural anaesthesia may be technically more difficult in the older patient, but there is no reason why it should be contraindicated.

C Hypotension secondary to sympathetic block can be complicated by the hypovolaemia of rapid blood loss.

D This is controversial: some think aspirin increases the risk of bleeding from the operation; some think it increases the risk of epidural haematoma; and some are wary of regional anaesthesia in a patient who has suffered transient ischaemic attacks. We have settled on 'false'; others might disagree. You should be prepared to discuss controversial topics in written papers or in vivas.

E An epidural is not contraindicated, but one would need caution if the patient was untreated, and an epidural in a beta-blocked patient could mask hypovolaemia until sudden cardiovascular collapse.

I.7 TTFTF

C Mannitol will reduce intracranial pressure, but will not suppress an epileptic focus.

E Hyperventilation is not useful in suppressing epileptic seizures, though may be used later to reduce intracranial pressure if cerebral oedema develops.

I.8 TTFTT

C The shock is likely to produce hypotension rather than hypertension.

I.9 TFFTF

A,B He will have lost stomach acid and will have a hypochloraemic alkalosis with hypokalaemia.

C Surgery should wait until rehydration and correction of any electrolyte disturbance.

D Some anaesthetists always give small children atropine, others do not think it necessary, but it is certainly 'reasonable'.

E This technique is perfectly reasonable, but some anaesthetists prefer to use a non-depolarising agent or an awake intubation technique.

I.10   TTTFF

 D   Ketamine maintains the laryngeal reflexes better than other agents, which makes aspiration less likely but does not prevent it.
 E   Diabetes is not a contraindication to ketamine. There would, if anything, be a slight increase in blood sugar due to catecholamine release.

I.11   FTFFT

Suxamethonium and d-tubocurarine are the two anaesthetic drugs most commonly associated with clinically important histamine release. Curare is now rarely used, but its historical importance means that questions will be asked about it for some years yet.

I.12   TTTFT

 D   The Sanders injector is only suitable for use with a rigid bronchoscope.
 E   This is a good technique but the appropriate catheter mount must be available.

I.13   TTTTT

 A   C6 is above the pleura – but there will only be 'no risk' if you can identify C6 accurately.
 E   The local anaesthetic will spread to the stellate ganglion at the C6 level.

I.14   TTTTT

I.15   TTFTT

 C   The hypoglossal nerve goes through the hypoglossal canal, above the occipital condyle.

I.16   **FTFTT**

A   The metabolic acidosis causes *hyper*kalaemia.
C   There will no longer be a tendency to *hyper*kalaemia if the transplant is effective, but hypokalaemia is not a feature.

I.17   **TTFFT**

C   U waves are a sign of *hypo*kalaemia.
D   ST depression is not a sign of hyperkalaemia.

I.18   **TTFTT**

C   There will be a raised central venous pressure in the tachycardia of heart failure, but tachycardia in itself has no consistent effect.
E   There are giant 'a' waves and cannon waves in tricuspid incompetence.

I.19   **TFFTT**

A,D,   Paroxysmal nocturnal dyspnoea is a feature of left-sided
E   heart failure.
C   Pulmonary stenosis causes relative pulmonary hypovolaemia, not congestion.

I.20   **TFFFF**

B   Blood pressure is unchanged.
D,E Hyperventilation and polyuria occur in *hyper*glycaemic coma: did you misread the question?

I.21   **TFFTF**

You will not need to know much dermatology, but its relevance in general medicine can be important.
B,C Hodgkin's disease and obstructive jaundice cause itch but no rash.
E   There is no itch in shingles. The rash is generalised only in the immunosuppressed.

I.22   FTFTT

Two typically 'opposite-option' answers: constipation occurs in **A** *hypo*kalaemia and **C** *hyper*calcaemia.

I.23   FFTTF

A   Relaxation occurs only if local anaesthetic is injected directly into muscle.

B   Suxamethonium may cause prolonged contraction.

C,D   The effects of non-depolarising drugs can be unpredictable.

E   The diaphragm may be affected.

I.24   TTFTT

C H_2-receptor antagonists are used for prophylaxis, but are not helpful in the treatment, of Mendelson's syndrome.

D   It is important that gastric carcinoma is excluded before H_2-receptor antagonists are prescribed.

I.25   TFFTF

B   Chronic pyelonephritis, unlike chronic glomerulonephritis, does not cause a large protein loss.

C   Fever is the presenting symptom in one fifth of cases.

E   Obviously infection must be eradicated before transplantation, but renal failure caused by chronic pyelonephritis is not a contraindication to transplantation.

I.26   FTFFF

The important word here is *severe*.

A   A right-sided pneumothorax will deviate the trachea somewhat to the right. A left-sided *tension* pneumothorax would probably cause more obvious deviation to the right.

C   Collapse of the left lung will move the trachea somewhat to the left.

D,E   Left-sided empyema or left pneumonectomy will probably move the trachea moderately to the left.

I.27   TTTFF

Not all patients show classical signs.

A,B   Don't be tricked into thinking that because these branches are worded the same they can't both be true: they are.

D   There is usually no definite relation between eating and pain in carcinoma of the stomach.

E   The pain of pyelonephritis may be felt around the flank but renal colic radiates to the groin.

I.28   FTFFT

You are given only a very brief clinical summary: the correct answers must reflect that.

A   There is nothing specific to suggest pyelonephritis.

B,C,   Swinging pyrexia suggests abscess: subphrenic or pelvic

E   are likely sites. A pleural effusion would be further evidence for a subphrenic abscess.

D   The problem could be a wound infection, which would not require a laparotomy. Treatment is initially expectant.

I.29   TTFFT

B   'Never' is uncommon in medicine. Nonetheless, chronic duodenal ulcers never become malignant (see Bailey & Love's *Short Practice of Surgery*, 21st edn. Lewis, London 1991).

C,E   Malignant change is uncommon in a chronic ulcer. 20% of prepyloric ulcers are malignant – that does not imply that they were all initially benign.

D   This was not true in the first edition of this book; it is even less true now.

I.30   TTTTT

There are other common causes of haematuria, and rare ones as well.

Paper II Questions

II.1 Likely causes of sudden death under anaesthesia include:
A   recent silent myocardial infarction
B   tight aortic stenosis
C   mitral incompetence
D   second-degree heart block
E   ventriculo-septal defect.

II.2 Appropriate anaesthetic techniques for microsurgery of the larynx include the use of:
A   a 5 mm endotracheal tube with low-volume, smooth profile cuff
B   neuroleptanaesthesia
C   apnoeic insufflation
D   Sanders injector
E   spontaneous ventilation.

II.3 End-tidal concentrations of carbon dioxide from a ventilated patient during anaesthesia using a circle absorption system:
A   are independent of fresh gas flow
B   are usually measured with an ultraviolet analyser
C   are independent of minute ventilation
D   are elevated by opioids
E   will decrease steadily in a semi-closed circle system incorporating soda lime.

II.4 Likely causes of postoperative confusion include:
A   hypoglycaemia
B   hypercapnia
C   uraemia
D   anaemia
E   incomplete neuromuscular reversal.

II.5   In the diagnosis of brain death:
A   criteria cannot be carried out in a spontaneously breathing patient
B   caloric testing is used to test the integrity of the Vth cranial nerve
C   serial 'flat' EEGs are required
D   the absence of neuromuscular blockade should be confirmed with a peripheral nerve stimulator
E   reflex movements of the legs may still occur.

II.6   Methods of reducing intracranial pressure before surgery include:
A   hyperventilation
B   sodium nitroprusside
C   spinal drainage
D   mannitol
E   propranolol.

II.7   Epidural analgesia in obstetric practice:
A   commonly causes itching
B   controls blood pressure in pre-eclampsia
C   causes uterine relaxation
D   can cause retention of urine
E   can contribute to the effects of caval compression.

II.8   In the very young:
A   the normal tidal volume of a 4 kg infant is 20–25 ml
B   the correct size of endotracheal tube in a 4-year-old child is likely to be 4.5 mm
C   the blood volume of a 7 kg infant is approximately 700 ml
D   the normal dose of neostigmine is 0.04–0.08 mg/kg
E   neonates tend to be sensitive to suxamethonium.

II.9   Halothane affects cardiovascular haemodynamics in the normocapnic patient by:
A   a direct myocardial effect
B   catecholamine release
C   a direct effect on the sinoatrial node
D   a peripheral vasodilatory effect
E   vagal depression.

II.10 **Following reversal of a non-depolarising muscle relaxant with neostigmine 2.5 mg and atropine 1.0 mg, a patient has difficulty breathing. There is tracheal tug, but no cyanosis when breathing supplementary oxygen. Correct treatment should include:**

A giving a further dose of reversal agents
B setting up a doxapram infusion
C testing the adequacy of neuromuscular transmission with a peripheral nerve stimulator
D direct laryngoscopy
E respiratory stimulation with carbon dioxide.

II.11 **The following are true of these laryngeal muscles and movements:**

A the posterior cricoarytenoids abduct the cords
B the lateral cricoarytenoids externally rotate the arytenoid cartilages
C the cricothyroid muscle tenses the cords
D there is no specific muscle that acts to relax the cords
E the cords are normally actively abducted in inspiration.

II.12 **The long saphenous vein:**

A courses from the medial side of the foot to the femoral vein just below the inguinal ligament
B lies just behind the medial malleolus
C lies behind the saphenous nerve in the lower leg
D has many communications with the deep veins of the leg
E is superficial for most of its course.

II.13 **The trigeminal nerve:**

A emerges from the brain at the level of the pons
B divides beyond the sphenopalatine ganglion into its ophthalmic, maxillary and mandibular branches
C innervates the lacrimal gland via the nasociliary branch of the ophthalmic division
D supplies sympathetic vasoconstrictor fibres to the eye
E does not innervate orbicularis oculi.

II.14 **The following statements about nerve supply are true:**

A the lateral popliteal nerve is more prone to damage than the medial popliteal
B damage to the sciatic nerve is a complication of posterior fracture-dislocation of the hip
C the pudendal nerve supplies the anal sphincter and perianal skin
D sciatic nerve block necessitates the patient being turned laterally or prone
E dorsiflexion of the great toe is from L4.

II.15 The following are true of water intoxication caused by overtransfusion with 5% dextrose:

A epileptiform convulsions are a recognised feature
B patients have muscle weakness
C the plasma sodium will be about 140 mmol/l
D it is essential to correct the total sodium deficit rapidly
E treatment should include hypertonic saline.

II.16 The following are true of the atypical ventricular tachycardia known as *torsades de pointes*:

A it is caused by hypomagnesaemia
B it is a side-effect of antiarrhythmic drugs
C the QRS complexes have a varying axis
D cardioversion is ineffective
E isoprenaline is a possible treatment.

II.17 Recognised effects of cardiac glycosides upon the electrocardiogram include:

A prolongation of the PR interval
B prolongation of the QT interval
C nodal rhythm
D ST depression
E tachycardia.

II.18 A high venous pressure, hypotension and acute circulatory failure occur in:

A tension pneumothorax
B pulmonary embolism
C congestive cardiac failure
D venous air embolism
E haemorrhage.

II.19 The following occur in primary myxoedema:

A bradycardia
B median nerve compression
C macrocytic anaemia
D flat T waves on the electrocardiogram
E hypertension.

II.20 Preoperative findings consistent with a diagnosis of phaeochromocytoma include:

A decreased haematocrit
B reduced plasma volume
C decreased serum sodium
D abnormal glucose tolerance test
E increased excretion of homovanillic acid.

II.21 **The following are likely diagnoses in a patient with jaundice and increased bilirubin in the urine:**
  A   infective hepatitis
  B   obstruction of the bile ducts
  C   liver disease caused by chlorpromazine
  D   metastatic carcinoma in the liver
  E   acute haemolysis.

II.22 **A 40-year-old female, admitted for elective hysterectomy, is found to have a haemoglobin of 8.2 g/dl and a reticulocyte count of 12%. This is compatible with a diagnosis of:**
  A   rheumatoid arthritis
  B   chronic renal failure
  C   menorrhagia
  D   myxoedema
  E   systemic lupus erythematosus.

II.23 **Flaccidity with extensor plantar responses occurs in:**
  A   motor neurone disease
  B   the acute phase of poliomyelitis
  C   the chronic phase of poliomyelitis
  D   Guillain–Barré syndrome
  E   syringomyelia.

II.24 **A urine specific gravity of 1030 occurs in:**
  A   diabetes insipidus
  B   impaired renal function
  C   dehydration
  D   diabetes mellitus
  E   total parenteral nutrition.

II.25 **Alveolar hyperventilation occurs in:**
  A   hypoxia
  B   respiratory acidosis
  C   salicylate overdose
  D   meningitis
  E   hypertension.

II.26 **In chronic bronchitis:**
  A   spirometric changes occur early
  B   clubbing is common
  C   chest radiography is usually normal
  D   steroids are usually ineffective
  E   the likeliest pathogen to cause acute exacerbation is *Haemophilus influenzae*.

II.27 Carcinoma of the pancreas:
  A   is commoner in males than females
  B   overall has a poor prognosis
  C   is likely to present earlier if it is in the head of the pancreas
  D   presents with diarrhoea
  E   can be cured by a Whipple's operation.

II.28 Indications for surgical correction of a sliding hiatus hernia include:
  A   anaemia
  B   a tendency to bronchospasm
  C   lung abscess
  D   peptic stricture
  E   associated pharyngeal pouch.

II.29 In a patient with a severe closed head injury:
  A   intracranial pressure is dependent upon mean arterial blood pressure
  B   intracranial pressure increases in direct proportion to the application of positive end-expiratory pressure (PEEP) to the airway
  C   fixed dilated pupils indicate severe cerebral injury
  D   treatment of choice includes hyperventilation to a $PaCO_2$ below 3.0 kPa (23 mmHg)
  E   leakage of cerebrospinal fluid must be stopped immediately.

II.30 When malignant hyperthermia occurs during anaesthesia:
  A   non-depolarising muscle relaxants are less effective than expected
  B   the body temperature increases about 1°C every 30 minutes
  C   there is severe metabolic acidosis
  D   serum potassium concentrations increase
  E   there is ventilatory failure.

Paper II Answers

II.1 **TTFFF**

  C,E Neither mitral incompetence nor ventriculo-septal defect is associated with sudden death under anaesthesia.

  D Second-degree heart block is not in itself an association. Some types of second-degree block predispose to complete heart block.

II.2 **FTTTT**

  There are many possible ways of giving anaesthesia for laryngeal microsurgery.

  A A microlaryngoscopy tube has a *high-volume*, low pressure cuff.

  B Neurolept drugs may be used to aid an 'awake' fibreoptic intubation.

  C This is insufflation with 100% oxygen into denitrogenated lungs. Carbon dioxide accumulates.

  D The Sanders injector relies on the Venturi effect to deliver a reasonable tidal volume.

II.3 **TFFFF**

  B CO_2 is analysed with *infrared* gas analysis.

  C $PetCO_2$ is inversely proportional to alveolar ventilation by *fresh* (which is CO_2-free) gas.

  D The patient is being ventilated so respiratory sensitivity to CO_2 is irrelevant: $PetCO_2$ may decrease because of a reduction in metabolic rate.

  E CO_2 concentrations will reach an equilibrium depending on the balance between metabolic rate and minute ventilation.

II.4 **TTTFF**

  A–C Many metabolic and biochemical disturbances are likely to cause postoperative confusion.

  D Anaemia, unless accompanied by severe hypoxia, will not cause confusion.

  E The patient may be distressed but is rarely confused unless other anaesthetic factors are also present.

II.5 TFFTT

A   A patient cannot be brain dead if breathing spontaneously. Ensure that you are aware of the difference between brain stem death and persistent vegetative state.

B   Caloric testing tests the VIIIth nerve.

C   EEGs are not part of the diagnosis in this country.

E   The limbs may move because of spinal reflexes.

II.6 TFFTT

B   Sodium nitroprusside, by causing vasodilation, increases intracranial pressure within the closed cranium.

C   If there is evidence of raised intracranial pressure on fundoscopy or CT scan, dural puncture is contraindicated because of the risk of coning.

II.7 TTFTT

A   Itching is commonest if opioids are added to the epidural mixture. At the time of writing their use is becoming more popular.

C   Epidural analgesia does not alter uterine tone, although it may reduce the spasm of discoordinated uterine contraction.

II.8 TFFTF

B   A formula is (age/4) + 4.5, which gives 5.5 mm. The likeliest size is 5.0–5.5; only a small 4-year-old would need a 4.5.

C   Neonates have a blood volume of 100 ml/kg, but this falls soon after birth to 85 ml/kg, which is 600 ml. The question says 'infant'.

E   Neonates are resistant to suxamethonium.

II.9 TFTTF

B   Halothane in a normocapnic patient is a sympathetic depressant.

E   Halothane, in common with many anaesthetic drugs, is vagotonic.

II.10   TFTTF

B   Doxapram is contraindicated in patients whose neuromuscular blockade is incompletely reversed.

C   It is reasonable to test neuromuscular stimulation once. A conscious patient will not thank you for repeatedly shocking them!

D   The presence of clot or a pedunculated polyp partly obstructing the airway may mimic the signs of incomplete reversal.

E   The patient may already be developing ventilatory failure and carbon dioxide will only make the situation worse.

II.11   TFTFT

B   The lateral cricoarytenoids adduct by internally rotating the arytenoid cartilages.

D   The thyroarytenoids relax the cords.

II.12   TFTTT

All these answers should be obvious to any anaesthetist who has kept their eyes open during surgery for varicose veins.

B   The long saphenous lies in front of the medial malleolus, an important site for venous access in fat infants and for cut-downs in severely shocked patients.

II.13   TFFFT

Take care with questions that contain a lot of detail: it must all be correct. Some people believe that multiple choice questions should not have 'conditional' branches. These are branches that are 'false' overall but contain a 'true' part. In general, we agree with this, but these 'double jeopardy' questions do get asked and you must learn to deal with them.

B   Here, the divisions are correct, but it is the wrong ganglion: it should be the trigeminal (Gasserian) not sphenopalatine.

C   The trigeminal *does* innervate the lacrimal gland, but via the lacrimal (not nasociliary) branch of the ophthalmic division.

D   The sympathetic vasoconstrictor fibres come from the superior cervical ganglion via the internal carotid plexus.

E   Orbicularis oculi is innervated by the facial nerve.

II.14   TTTFT

C   The innervation is from the pudendal nerve via the inferior rectal nerve.

D   The sciatic nerve can be blocked by an anterior approach in the upper thigh.

E   This innervation is useful when testing for the level of root lesions.

II.15 TTFFT

C,D The wording of these two branches is to suggest that while total sodium is low, plasma sodium is maintained. This is not so. Plasma sodium will be very low (<120 mmol/l). Urine osmolarity will also be low, with maximally dilute urine (SG = 1.001).

D Rapid correction of the sodium deficit may cause permanent brain damage. Women of childbearing age are especially at risk.

E Water restriction may be enough, but hypertonic saline is recommended in severe cases.

II.16 TTTFT

A *Torsades de pointes* can be caused by hypomagnesaemia, hypokalaemia or hypocalcaemia.

B Type I antiarrhythmic drugs can precipitate the condition, and should not be used to treat it.

D Cardioversion is a reasonable treatment.

II.17 TFTTF

B,E Digoxin shortens the QT interval and reduces the heart rate.

II.18 TTTFF

D,E Air embolism and haemorrhage cause acute circulatory failure and hypotension, but central venous pressure is low.

II.19 TTTTF

C Macrocytic anaemia is usually thought to be associated with the development of pernicious anaemia.

E There is usually hypotension.

II.20 FTFTT

A,B These two are mutually exclusive – plasma volume is decreased and so haematocrit must increase unless there is concomitant anaemia – which there is not in phaeochromocytoma.

C Serum sodium is not abnormal.

II.21   TTTTF

It is important to learn the various permutations of what goes up and what goes down in jaundice of varying causation.

A–D   Any degree of obstruction will raise the urinary bilirubin. Chlorpromazine causes a cholestatic jaundice.

II.22   TTTFT

D   In myxoedema the haemoglobin would probably be higher than 8 g/dl, and the reticulocyte count would be normal.

II.23   TFFFT

A   Motor neurone disease is the most common cause of flaccidity with extensor plantar responses.

B–D   Poliomyelitis and Guillain–Barré syndrome cause flaccidity only.

E   The combination is rare in syringomyelia.

II.24   FFTTT

A   In diabetes insipidus there is a high urine volume of low specific gravity.

B   If renal function is impaired, the kidneys cannot concentrate urine.

II.25   TFTTF

B   Respiratory acidosis is, by definition, acidosis secondary to hypoventilation. If there is massive ventilation/perfusion imbalance, the carbon dioxide will be raised despite hyperventilation, but that is stretching a point: the answer to this branch is 'false'.

E   Not with hypertension, but hypotension may cause hyperventilation.

II.26   FFTTT

A   The usual spirometric tests (e.g. peak flow and forced expiratory volumes) are unchanged in chronic bronchitis until there is already a considerable degree of obstruction of the smallest airways.

B   Clubbing is rare and is an alerting sign to check for bronchogenic carcinoma.

D   It may be worth giving steroids a trial.

II.27   **TTTTT**

A   Carcinoma of the pancreas is slightly more common in males.

C   About 70% of cases are in the head of the pancreas; the earlier presentation is because the tumour compresses the common bile duct and causes early jaundice.

D   Diarrhoea is not the commonest presentation but is often a symptom.

E   Whipple's operation is theoretically curative but isn't always effective: the 5-year survival after resection of a periampullary tumour is perhaps better than 30%.

II.28   **TTTTF**

A   The implication is that the anaemia is secondary to bleeding from mucosa involved in the hernia.

B,C   Bronchospasm increases the likelihood of aspiration.

E   Pharyngeal pouches occur at the other end of the oesophagus and have no association with hiatus hernia.

II.29   **TFFFF**

B   The intracranial pressure will increase with application of pressure to the airway, secondary to an increase in venous pressure and a decrease in the cerebral compliance, but there is no direct simple relation between the two pressures.

C   Fixed dilated pupils can be a sign of bilateral damage to the oculomotor nerves.

D   Extreme hyperventilation is not indicated.

E   Cerebrospinal fluid leak does not need to be stopped *immediately*.

II.30   **TTTTF**

E   There will be hyperventilation in response to the metabolic acidosis.

Paper III Questions

III.1 **Appropriate agents for use during synchronised electrical reversal of atrial arrhythmias include:**
  A midazolam
  B etomidate
  C mivacurium
  D thiopentone
  E methohexitone.

III.2 **Indications for general anaesthesia for dental surgery include:**
  A mental retardation
  B infection near the site of surgery
  C porphyria
  D pregnancy
  E removal of four wisdom teeth.

III.3 **The following are true of the sterilisation of anaesthetic equipment:**
  A boiling in water for 15 minutes at atmospheric pressure kills bacterial spores
  B an autoclave pressure of 1 bar at a temperature of 120°C for 15 minutes kills all living organisms
  C gamma irradiation is an effective means of sterilisation
  D ethylene oxide takes 2 hours to be completely effective
  E a solution of chlorhexidine sterilises an endotracheal tube in 3 minutes.

III.4 **The following are true of reflex activity during anaesthesia:**
  A the gag reflex is abolished in plane 2 of stage 3
  B carinal stimulation will induce coughing during surgical anaesthesia above stage 4
  C anal dilation will produce laryngospasm in stage 3
  D traction on the external ocular muscles commonly produces tachycardia
  E tracheal tug is a reflex response to intercostal paralysis.

III.5 **Perioperative haemorrhage in a patient with haemophilia undergoing emergency surgery can be treated by the following, alone or in combination:**
A   transfusion of SAG-M blood
B   transfusion of fresh frozen plasma
C   factor VIII concentrate
D   aprotinin
E   platelet concentrate.

III.6 **In the casualty department, a 45-year-old man falls to the ground. You can feel no pulse. You should immediately:**
A   await recovery from a vaso-vagal attack
B   check that the airway is clear
C   give a precordial thump
D   ventilate the patient by facemask
E   apply defibrillation.

III.7 **The following are true of general anaesthesia for caesarean section:**
A   general anaesthesia reduces gastric pH
B   MAC is increased
C   it is contraindicated in patients with a bleeding diathesis
D   it is a major cause of maternal mortality
E   atracurium causes histamine release in the fetus.

III.8 **Appropriate techniques in the treatment of eclampsia include:**
A   intravenous labetalol
B   lumbar epidural anaesthesia
C   intravenous magnesium sulphate
D   intravenous phenytoin
E   rehydration with salt-free fluids.

III.9   **Pupillary constriction during anaesthesia is produced by:**
A   sodium nitroprusside
B   surgical stimulus
C   naloxone
D   fentanyl
E   dopamine.

III.10   **The following drugs have interactions with drugs commonly used during anaesthesia:**
A   imipramine
B   chlordiazepoxide
C   phenelzine
D   interferon
E   levodopa.

III.11   **Factors likely to contribute to the development of postoperative hepatic failure include:**
A   hypertension
B   hypoxia
C   blood transfusion
D   hypercapnia
E   septicaemia.

III.12   **After left lower lobectomy:**
A   underwater apical and basal chest drains are inserted
B   mediastinal flap occurs
C   the left heart border is no longer seen on the chest radiograph
D   atrial fibrillation is a recognised complication
E   there is increased risk of staphylococcal pneumonia.

III.13   **The skin over the occiput and the back of the neck is supplied by:**
A   a branch of the first cervical nerve
B   the medial branch of the second cervical nerve
C   the greater occipital nerve
D   overlap from the lesser occipital nerve
E   the medial branches of C6–8.

III.14   The following are true of the arteries at the base of the brain:
A   the internal carotid eventually becomes the middle cerebral
B   the anterior communicating is the anterior anastomotic connection between the internal carotid systems
C   the posterior communicating arteries join the internal carotids to the basilar
D   the posterior communicating arteries are absent in 12–18% of the population
E   the internal carotid lies lateral to the optic nerve.

III.15   Femoral nerve block:
A   reduces the pain of a fractured neck of femur
B   is part of the field block for repair of a femoral hernia
C   is blocked medial to the femoral artery just below the inguinal ligament
D   permits operations on the patella
E   is contraindicated if there is peripheral vascular disease of the leg.

III.16   A blood urea concentration of 13 mmol/l occurs in:
A   dehydration
B   gastrointestinal haemorrhage
C   pyloric stenosis in a boy aged 5 weeks
D   congestive cardiac failure
E   water intoxication.

III.17   Causes of cardiomyopathy include:
A   thyrotoxicosis
B   porphyria
C   dystrophia myotonica
D   alcoholism
E   prolonged artificial ventilation.

III.18   In a patient with severe arteriosclerosis:
A   autoregulation of renal blood flow is impaired
B   angiotensin-converting enzyme (ACE) inhibitors are the antihypertensives of choice
C   droperidol is contraindicated
D   preoperative treatment with beta-adrenergic blocking drugs should be discontinued at least 24 hours preoperatively
E   induced hypotension is contraindicated.

III.19 **In partial right bundle branch block (RBBB):**
A   the QRS complex is wider than normal
B   S waves are slurred in leads I, V5 and V6
C   there is ST depression in chest leads V1 and V2
D   there is T wave inversion in leads V1 and V2
E   P waves are inverted.

III.20 **Symptoms of a thyroid crisis include:**
A   fever
B   bronchospasm
C   abdominal pain
D   cardiac arrhythmias
E   coma.

III.21 **Complications of diverticular disease likely to require surgical intervention include:**
A   haemorrhage
B   vesicovaginal fistula
C   stricture formation
D   small bowel obstruction
E   anaemia.

III.22 **In a patient with chronic hepatic disease:**
A   the action of suxamethonium is prolonged
B   metabolism of opioids is delayed
C   vitamin K absorption is reduced
D   prothrombin time is prolonged
E   dosage of non-depolarising neuromuscular blocking drugs should be reduced.

III.23 **Eaton–Lambert (myasthenic) syndrome:**
A   is a complication of bronchogenic carcinoma
B   affects similar muscle groups to myasthenia gravis
C   causes diminished tendon reflexes
D   is helped by intravenous anticholinesterases
E   is improved by thymectomy.

III.24 **Drugs that can cause jaundice include:**
A   methyldopa
B   chlorpromazine
C   isoflurane
D   diazepam
E   isoniazid.

III.25   The following are features of chronic renal failure:
A   bleeding tendency
B   macrocytic anaemia
C   hypertension
D   splenomegaly
E   lassitude.

III.26   Causes of haemoptysis include:
A   Goodpasture's syndrome
B   bronchiectasis
C   mitral stenosis
D   pulmonary embolism
E   Mallory–Weiss syndrome.

III.27   A 60-year-old man complains of acute abdominal pain after a proven anterolateral myocardial infarction. The systolic blood pressure is 80 mmHg, bowel sounds are absent and the abdomen is distended. Likely diagnoses include:
A   acute cholecystitis
B   superior mesenteric artery embolism
C   diverticulitis of sigmoid colon
D   acute pancreatitis
E   perforated peptic ulcer.

III.28   After splenectomy:
A   there is an initial leucocytosis
B   an initial phase of hypocoagulability is followed by hypercoagulability
C   there is an increased risk of pneumococcal pneumonia
D   there is an increased incidence of portal hypertension
E   maximal exercise tolerance is reduced.

III.29   In the differential diagnosis between diverticulitis and carcinoma of the colon, the following would favour diverticulitis:
A   weight loss
B   abdominal pain
C   episodes of profuse bleeding
D   a palpable mass in the left iliac fossa
E   a long history.

III.30 Dislocation of the shoulder:
  A   usually displaces anteriorly
  B   usually prevents the patient using the arm at all
  C   can paralyse the deltoid muscle
  D   requires general anaesthesia for reduction
  E   if recurrent, tends to occur on external rotation.

Paper III Answers

III.1 TTFTT

C Suxamethonium might be used to permit a rapid sequence intubation, but a non-depolarising agent has a slower onset time and (usually) an unnecessarily long duration of action for this procedure.

III.2 TTFFF

A These patients are often too difficult for local anaesthesia.
B Local anaesthesia does not work well when there is infection.
C,D These are relative contraindications to *general* anaesthesia, whether in the dental chair or not.
E Anaesthetists see a lot of these cases, but many more are done without the need for general anaesthetic – although only two teeth can be removed at one local anaesthetic session.

III.3 FTTFF

A Boiling in water for 15 minutes at atmospheric pressure will kill only bacteria, not bacterial spores.
D Ethylene oxide needs 10–12 hours for full effect. It is extremely toxic and apparatus must then be thoroughly aerated.
E An endotracheal tube needs 20 minutes in chlorhexidine (0.1%).

III.4 TTTFF

D Pulling on the external ocular muscles causes bradycardia by vagal stimulation.
E Tracheal tug is caused by an increased pressure difference between the atmosphere and the thorax. This pressure difference is exaggerated by airway obstruction, when tug is especially obvious. Tug is also seen when breathing is diaphragmatic, in deeply anaesthetised but not necessarily obstructed patients. It is not a reflex: the muscles of the upper airway and the accessory muscles of breathing are also paralysed by that stage.

III.5 **TTTFF**

  A SAG-M blood contains no clotting factors, but this is the commonest way of replacing red cells.

  B,C Fresh frozen plasma contains too low a concentration of clotting factors to be total treatment, but factor VIII may not be immediately available.

  D Aprotinin enhances platelet activity.

  E Platelets are no use in haemophilia, unless massive transfusion has caused a dilutional thrombocytopenia. Platelets may be helpful in von Willebrand's disease.

III.6 **FTTTF**

  A Basic life support measures should be started. If the patient has fainted, the measures are still needed and effective. If the patient has an arrhythmia, no time has been wasted.

  C,E A precordial thump is now recommended early in advanced resuscitation. Defibrillation is indicated only if VF is present, which requires diagnosis of the rhythm and is excluded in this question by the word 'immediately'.

III.7 **FFFFF**

  A General anaesthesia has no known effect on the gastric pH; the pH is low for other reasons.

  B Awareness in caesarean section occurred because anaesthetists were worried about the effect of anaesthetic vapours on the fetus. MAC is not noticeably altered by pregnancy.

  C The bleeding diathesis should be treated if possible: epidural and intrathecal anaesthesia are contraindicated.

  D Although important to anaesthetists, maternal mortality associated directly with anaesthesia is now only a small proportion of maternal deaths.

  E Atracurium is probably the best non-depolariser for caesarean section. It is ionised and crosses the placenta poorly. We don't suppose that anyone knows whether histamine release occurs in the fetus, but sometimes clinical judgement means deciding that something really is very unlikely. You shouldn't guess in MCQs, but marking this question 'don't know' suggests timidity.

III.8 **TTTTF**

  The treatment of eclampsia undergoes periodic shifts. At the time of writing **A–D** are regarded as useful.

  E The circulating blood volume is reduced in eclampsia and cautious re-expansion may be beneficial, but not with water.

III.9   FFFTF

A   Ganglion blockers dilate the pupils; nitroprusside has no effect.
B   Surgical stimulus causes pupillary dilation.
C   Naloxone reverses opioid-induced miosis.
E   Dopamine has no effect.

III.10   FFTFT

A   Imipramine is a tricyclic antidepressant, which has no important interactions with drugs used in general anaesthesia. Its important interactions are with cardiovascularly active drugs.
C   Phenelzine is a monoamine oxidase inhibitor.
D   Interferon is used in some malignancies and experimentally in a number of other diseases. It has no known interactions with anaesthetic drugs.
E   Levodopa is converted to dopamine in the basal ganglia, and there is a risk of dysrhythmias, especially with halothane. There may also be interaction with droperidol, which is a central dopamine antagonist.

III.11   FTTTT

Postoperative hepatic failure is exceedingly rare and is likely to occur only in patients with pre-existing hepatic dysfunction. Everyone knows about halothane hepatitis, but even that is rare – and becoming even less likely as usage of halothane decreases.
A   Hypotension predisposes to impaired hepatic perfusion and oxygenation.

III.12   TFFTF

B   Mediastinal flap is prevented by full expansion of the other lung.
C   The left heart border will be visible provided that the remaining (upper) lobe is expanded.
E   Postoperative chest infection is a risk of thoracic surgery, but there is no special risk of staphylococcal pneumonia.

III.13   FTTTF

The general pattern of afferent innervation is from the medial branches of the posterior primary rami; the lateral branches are normally motor. C1 is motor only.
C   C2: the largest posterior primary ramus.
D   There is overlap anteriorly, via the cervical plexus, with the lesser occipital nerve, which is a branch of the anterior primary ramus.
E   C3–5 supply the posterior skin; C6–8 do not.

III.14 **TTFFT**

A   The internal carotid becomes the anterior cerebral and then the middle cerebral.

C   The posterior communicating arteries are the anastomotic connections between the areas of supply of the internal carotids and the basilars, but the arteries actually join the internal carotids to the posterior cerebrals.

D   Absence of posterior communicating arteries is not a recognised anomaly.

III.15 **TFFFF**

B   There is no femoral distribution this proximal.

C   The femoral nerve is *lateral* to the artery.

D   Analgesia of the patella requires block of the femoral, obturator and lateral cutaneous nerve of thigh.

E   Blocks are especially suitable for patients with vascular disease, though solutions containing vasoconstrictors are better avoided, especially for ankle blocks.

III.16 **TTFTF**

B   Absorption and subsequent breakdown of haemoglobin increases the plasma urea.

C   Pyloric stenosis causes a metabolic alkalosis, but not uraemia.

D   A reasonably likely result, because of reduced renal perfusion caused by low cardiac output.

III.17 **TTTTF**

D   Alcohol causes a primary cardiomyopathy; the other causes here are secondary. The distinction is not as important as the recognition that cardiomyopathy occurs.

E   There is no described association between prolonged ventilation and cardiomyopathy.

III.18 **TFFFT**

B   Studies suggest that ACE inhibitors are the treatment of choice *for patients in cardiac failure*; their use in arteriosclerosis is not defined at the time of writing.

C   Droperidol in normal anaesthetic dosage is cardiovascularly stable.

D   Antihypertensive therapy should be maintained up to, and after, the time of operation.

E   Large decreases in blood pressure may compromise the cerebral or coronary circulation.

III.19   FTTTF

A   The QRS complex is wide in complete RBBB. The QRS is wide in partial LBBB.

E   Atrial conduction is unaffected.

III.20   TFTTT

B   Bronchospasm is not a feature of thyroid crisis.

III.21   TTTTF

E   Anaemia is a common complication of diverticular disease but is not an indication for operation.

III.22   FTFTF

A   The action of suxamethonium is prolonged only if there is severe hepatic failure, not if a patient has stable chronic disease.

C   Vitamin K absorption is reduced in jaundice.

E   In the first edition the answer was 'true', but the modern non-depolarising relaxants cause fewer problems. Atracurium and mivacurium have alternative pathways of metabolism, which include pseudocholinesterase: thus if **A** is false, so is **E**.

III.23   TFTFF

Eaton–Lambert syndrome is a peripheral myasthenia occurring in about 1% of patients with oat cell carcinoma and occurs rarely in association with other tumours.

B   Eaton–Lambert syndrome causes predominantly peripheral muscular weakness.

D   Intravenous anticholinesterases do not improve the weakness.

E   Thymectomy is an operation for myasthenia gravis. It has no place in myasthenic syndrome. The weakness of the syndrome may improve if the primary tumour is resected.

III.24   TTFFT

C   At the time of writing, there is no established link between isoflurane and hepatic damage.

III.25   TFTFT

    B   Chronic renal failure causes a microcytic anaemia.

III.26   FTTTF

Do not worry if you had not heard of Goodpasture's syndrome or Mallory–Weiss syndrome – *unless you guessed and got them wrong.* You should have known that bronchiectasis and mitral stenosis cause haemoptysis.

    A   Goodpasture's syndrome is pulmonary haemorrhage associated with proliferative glomerulonephritis.

    D   Uncomplicated pulmonary embolus does not cause haemoptysis, but embolus into a damaged lung – for example in a patient with chronic lung disease – can cause infarction of the distal lung.

    E   Mallory–Weiss syndrome may mimic haemoptysis, but is caused by persistent vomiting.

III.27   FTFFT

This is a clinical scenario question. In the examination room, cover up the branches and work out what might be going on before looking at them.

The key words are 'proven' myocardial infarction and 'likely' diagnoses. The most likely diagnosis is therefore **B** – superior mesenteric artery embolus. Of the others, only **E** is likely (the stress of an infarct can provoke ulceration). The other diagnoses are part of the differential diagnosis of the acute abdomen, but there is nothing to make them likely here.

III.28   TFTFF

    B   There is no phase of hypocoagulability. There is an increased platelet count and hypercoagulability.

    E   The spleen does not hold an important reserve of blood in humans and the oxygen-combining characteristics of haemoglobin and the red cells are unchanged by splenectomy.

III.29   FTTFT

    A   Weight loss makes a cancer more likely.

    C   Bleeding from carcinoma is usually in small amounts.

    D   A mass may be palpable in both conditions (which may anyway coexist); a tender mass favours diverticulitis.

III.30   TTTFT

B   Pain usually prevents movement after dislocating the shoulder.

C   The circumflex nerve can be damaged.

D   Reduction is often possible with sedation and analgesia. Interscalene block of the brachial plexus is another technique.

Paper IV Questions

IV.1 **Drugs which can safely be used when anaesthetising a patient at risk of development of malignant hyperpyrexia (MH) include:**
A lignocaine
B atropine
C droperidol
D enflurane
E suxamethonium.

IV.2 **During induction of anaesthesia in a patient with a quinsy:**
A the patient should be preoxygenated
B anaesthesia must be induced using a volatile agent
C suxamethonium is indicated to allow rapid intubation
D nasal intubation is contraindicated
E trismus relaxes with the onset of anaesthesia.

IV.3 **The following will precipitate a sickle cell crisis in a susceptible patient:**
A hypoxia
B hypercapnia
C hypotension
D alkalosis
E hypothermia.

IV.4 **Factors associated with the development of postoperative atelectasis include:**
A allowing the patient to breathe spontaneously during anaesthesia
B emphysema
C thoracic epidural for pain relief
D urinary retention
E spinal anaesthesia.

IV.5 Measures commonly used in the treatment of Gram-negative septicaemia include:

A   beta-adrenergic blockade
B   the transfusion of fresh frozen plasma
C   inotropic support by phosphodiesterase inhibitors
D   alpha-adrenergic blockade
E   intravenous heparin.

IV.6 Side-effects of opioid drugs that limit their use for postoperative neurosurgical patients include:

A   respiratory depression
B   interference with pupillary responses
C   depression of the cough reflex
D   causing euphoria
E   constipation.

IV.7 Placental blood flow is:

A   independent of mean arterial blood pressure
B   locally autoregulated
C   reduced in hypoxia
D   reduced by enflurane
E   increased by isoflurane.

IV.8 Suitable intravenous doses of drugs for use during anaesthesia in a 3-year-old child include:

A   neostigmine 0.08 mg/kg
B   atropine 0.02 mg/kg
C   trimeprazine 2 mg/kg
D   vecuronium 0.1 mg/kg
E   morphine 0.4 mg/kg.

IV.9 Non-depolarising neuromuscular blocking drugs are:

A   potentiated by edrophonium
B   sometimes ineffective in renal failure
C   usable with caution in myasthenia gravis
D   reversed by physostigmine
E   potentiated by hyponatraemia.

IV.10 **A low level of serum cholinesterase is caused by:**
A   hepatic disease
B   albuminuria
C   changes in the third trimester of pregnancy
D   cardiac failure
E   extensive procaine infiltration for local anaesthesia.

IV.11 **During one lung anaesthesia:**
A   inspired oxygen concentrations should be at least 50%
B   hyperoxic shunting reduces PaO_2
C CO_2 production is increased
D   airway pressure increases
E   dialled concentration of volatile anaesthetic should be doubled.

IV.12 **Local anaesthetic block of the ulnar nerve at the elbow:**
A   has a high incidence of postoperative neuritis
B   gives anaesthesia of the ulnar aspect of the forearm and hand
C   will miss the posterior division
D   will not affect grip
E   will not reliably give anaesthesia of the ring finger (fourth digit).

IV.13 **The following are true of the 'typical' vertebra:**
A   the pattern is that of the midthoracic vertebra
B   the spinal canal is bounded posteriorly by the laminae
C   the rib tubercles articulate with the transverse processes
D   the rib heads articulate with the vertebral bodies
E   the segmental nerves emerge below the corresponding vertebra.

IV.14 **The inferior dental nerve:**
A   is a pure sensory nerve
B   is blocked as it enters the mandibular foramen above and behind the third molar
C   when blocked, will give anaesthesia of all the ipsilateral lower teeth
D   successful block is likely to give partial anaesthesia of the tongue
E   ends by supplying sensation to the skin of the lower lip.

IV.15   The following are true of the brachial plexus:

A   it is primarily a plexus of sensory nerves
B   the cords are named from their relation to the axillary artery
C   there can be contributions from C4 and T2
D   anomalous cervical supply is often associated with anomalies of the first rib
E   block at the level of the first rib gives better anaesthesia in the radial distribution than the axillary approach.

IV.16: The following occur in water retention:

A   an increase in the central venous pressure
B   inappropriate concentration of urine
C   an increase in body weight
D   hypernatraemia
E   a plasma osmolarity of 310 mosmol/l.

IV.17   Causes of sinus tachycardia include:

A   thyrotoxicosis
B   constrictive pericarditis
C   anaemia
D   raised intracranial pressure
E   anxiety.

IV.18   A 40-year-old woman complains of increasing dyspnoea over 5 years. At cardiac catheterisation she has a systemic arterial pressure of 110/70 mmHg, a pulmonary artery pressure of 80/40 mmHg, a right atrial pressure of 5 mmHg, a pulmonary capillary wedge pressure of 9 mmHg, a right ventricular pressure of 80/5 mmHg and a left ventricular pressure of 110/8 mmHg. These results are compatible with a diagnosis of:

A   mitral stenosis
B   constrictive pericarditis
C   mitral insufficiency
D   primary myocardial disease
E   idiopathic pulmonary hypertension.

IV.19 A 40-year-old woman is to undergo routine cholecystectomy. She takes mesalazine (5-ASA) and rectal prednisolone for ulcerative colitis. The following are true:
 A ulcerative colitis is a factor in the development of gallstones
 B steroid therapy is a factor in the development of gallstones
 C she should be given hydrocortisone with her premedication
 D she should be given hydrocortisone 6 hours postoperatively
 E potassium should be added to her postoperative intravenous fluids.

IV.20 Generalised lymphadenopathy occurs in:
 A rubella
 B tuberculosis
 C Still's disease
 D disseminated lupus erythematosus
 E sarcoidosis.

IV.21 Persistent vomiting occurs in:
 A acute pancreatitis
 B intussusception
 C uraemia
 D increased intracranial pressure
 E hiatus hernia.

IV.22 Causes of iron-deficiency anaemia include:
 A rheumatoid arthritis
 B haemorrhage
 C uraemia
 D malabsorption
 E thalassaemia.

IV.23 The cardinal symptoms and signs of raised intracranial pressure include:
 A loss of peripheral vision
 B vomiting
 C papilloedema
 D vertigo with vertical nystagmus
 E a change of mental state.

IV.24   In renal ischaemia:

A   urine volume is increased
B   urinary sodium is decreased
C   urinary creatinine is decreased
D   the renal medulla is more at risk than the cortex
E   dobutamine selectively improves urine output.

IV.25   Mechanical ventilation during anaesthesia to a $PaCO_2$ of 3.5 kPa (26 mmHg) causes:

A   reduced cardiac output
B   vasoconstriction of skeletal muscle vessels
C   pupillary constriction
D   leftward shift of the oxyhaemoglobin dissociation curve
E   tissue hypoxia.

IV.26   The following signs are likely in a patient with an acute exacerbation of chronic bronchitis:

A   muscle twitching
B   papilloedema
C   reduced pulse pressure
D   confusion
E   pursed lips.

IV.27   Complications particularly associated with laparoscopic cholecystectomy include:

A   haemorrhage
B   division of the common bile duct
C   tension pneumothorax
D   persistent right hypochondrial pain
E   septicaemia.

IV.28 **Clinical features of small bowel obstruction include:**
A   constant central abdominal pain
B   nausea and vomiting
C   dullness to percussion in the flanks
D   abdominal distension
E   absent bowel sounds.

IV.29 **The following are true of acute pancreatitis:**
A   the acute phase usually follows 2–3 weeks of prodromal symptoms
B   fluid restriction is advisable in the early stages
C   the patient may need repeated calcium supplements
D   most patients develop hyperglycaemia
E   pancreatic pseudocyst is a rare complication.

IV.30 **After uretero-colic anastomosis:**
A   osteomalacia is a feature
B   there is a hyperchloraemic acidosis
C   patients should take extra salt
D   there is hypokalaemia
E   pyelonephritis is rare.

Paper IV Answers

IV.1 TTTFF

A No local anaesthetic is a trigger of MH.
C Some anaesthetists avoid phenothiazines and butyrophenones because of their association with the neuroleptic malignant syndrome, but there is no evidence that this syndrome is related to MH.
D All anaesthetic vapours should be avoided.
E Suxamethonium is a potent trigger.

IV.2 TFFFF

A Oxygen is always a good idea.
B A gaseous induction is not essential; an awake fibreoptic technique is an option. Remember that some quinsys are operable using local anaesthesia.
C Muscle relaxants of any type must be used extremely cautiously, and then only by anaesthetists with experience, in potential obstruction of the upper airway.
D Nasal intubation is the route of choice.
E Trismus usually relaxes, but it is a brave (or foolish) anaesthetist who relies on this: not all intraoral swellings are what they seem.

IV.3 TTTFT

D A crisis is precipitated by *acidosis*. Precipitating factors are related to impaired cellular oxygenation.

IV.4 FTFFF

A Basal atelectasis develops during general anaesthesia, whether the patient breathes spontaneously or is ventilated.
C Good pain relief allows the patient to take deeper breaths and reduces the incidence of atelectasis.
D There is no association between urinary retention and atelectasis.
E There is said to be a lesser incidence of pulmonary problems after spinal than after general anaesthesia.

IV.5 FFFFF

B,E The question states 'Gram-negative septicaemia', not multiorgan failure. Certainly, some patients who develop septicaemia eventually develop clotting problems as well, but the common primary problem is hypotension.

C Phosphodiesterase inhibitors cause peripheral vasodilation, which is not helpful in septicaemia (see **D**).

D The answer to this question in the last edition was 'true': vasodilation (with adequate infusion of fluid). The current vogue is to use noradrenaline to increase peripheral resistance in septicaemia with high cardiac output: times and fashions change – often on the basis of opinion rather than evidence.

IV.6 TTTFF

D Euphoria is not common after opioids, but might not be such a bad thing after major surgery!

E This is a side-effect of opioids, but not one that limits use after neurosurgery.

IV.7 FFTTF

A Placental blood flow is reduced in hypotension.

B There is no autoregulation.

D Any drug that reduces cardiac output will reduce placental flow.

E Vessels in the pregnant uterus are dilated already; a vasodilator has little effect.

IV.8 TTFTF

C Careful – the dose is correct, but trimeprazine is not given intravenously.

E Morphine 0.2 mg/kg is the usual quoted dose.

IV.9 FFTTF

A,D Edrophonium and physostigmine are both anticholinesterases.

B If affected at all by changes in renal function, neuromuscular blocking agents will be potentiated because of reduced excretion.

E There are theoretical effects of ionic imbalances on the action of these drugs, but the only one that matters clinically is the muscular weakness of hypokalaemia.

IV.10   TFTTF

B   Serum cholinesterase levels are not reduced by albuminuria.

E   This local anaesthetic is now rarely used, but is currently still in the BNF. It is metabolised by plasma cholinesterase, but does not affect the levels of the enzyme.

IV.11   FTFTF

A   Inspired oxygen concentration should be adjusted according to the individual patient's lung function and pulse oximetry.

C CO_2 production depends upon metabolism, not ventilation.

D   Compliance decreases and airway pressure increases unless tidal volume is decreased.

E   The concentration of volatile agent should be increased if the requirements for oxygenation mean the inspired nitrous oxide is reduced. Otherwise there is no need to adjust the concentration: there is an increase in shunt, not dead space, when only one lung is ventilated.

IV.12   TFFFT

A   The incidence of neuritis is high, especially in children.

B   The ulnar (medial) aspect of the forearm is supplied by cutaneous branches from the medial cord.

C   There are no branches of the ulnar nerve above the elbow.

D   The ulnar nerve supplies many of the small muscles of the hand.

E   There is individual variation of median and ulnar nerve supply to the ring finger.

IV.13   TTTTT

E   The cervical nerves emerge above the vertebra, but they are not 'typical'.

IV.14   FTTTT

A   The inferior dental nerve supplies muscles in the floor of the mouth before it enters the mandibular foramen.

D   The nerve does not innervate the tongue, but the lingual nerve lies close to the site of injection.

E   The nerve ends as the mental nerve.

IV.15 FTTTT
    A   There is no separation of motor and sensory fibres.

IV.16 FTTFF
    A   The central venous pressure will not increase in simple water retention.
    D,E There will be hyponatraemia and a reduced plasma osmolarity.

IV.17 TTTFT
    D   Raised intracranial pressure causes bradycardia.

IV.18 FFFFT
    A–D Pressures are normal in the atria, the left ventricle and the aorta: the only abnormal findings are hypertension in the right ventricle and pulmonary artery.

IV.19   FFTTF

A,B   There is no causative connection between ulcerative colitis or steroid therapy and gallstones.

C,D   Although rectal prednisolone rarely causes adrenal suppression, most texts suggest steroid cover if the patient has taken steroids at sufficient dosage for 2 months in the previous 6.

E   There is no special need for potassium.

IV.20   TTTTT

C   Still's disease is juvenile rheumatoid arthritis.

D   45% of patients with disseminated lupus erythematosus have generalised lymphadenopathy.

IV.21   TTTTF

E   In hiatus hernia there is usually regurgitation. There may be intermittent vomiting, but persistent vomiting is unusual.

IV.22   FTFTF

A,C,   Rheumatoid arthritis, uraemia and thalassaemia may
E   produce a hypochromic anaemia, but it is not iron-deficient and is more commonly normochromic.

IV.23   FTTFT

The cardinal features of raised intracranial pressure are vomiting (**B**), morning headaches, bradycardia, papilloedema (**C**) and a change of mental state (**E**). That is not to say that someone with increased pressure cannot have loss of vision or vertigo, but these are localising signs.

IV.24   FTTTF

A   Urine volume is decreased in renal ischaemia.

D   Although the kidney has a high total oxygen supply, the renal medulla is highly metabolically active and is more easily damaged by ischaemia.

E   Dopamine is the selective agent. Dobutamine increases urine output by increasing cardiac output. (Some people do not believe that even dopamine has a specific action on the kidney.)

IV.25   TTFTF

A   Other things being equal, hypocapnia reflexly reduces cardiac output.

B   All vascular smooth muscle is sensitive to local tissue tensions of carbon dioxide. Blood vessels in skeletal muscle will be vasoconstricted in an anaesthetised patient.

C   There is no direct effect of carbon dioxide on the pupils. If a patient is lightly anaesthetised and aware, over-ventilation can constrict the pupils because hypocapnia reduces the general level of arousal.

D,E   The left shift of the curve by this level of hypocapnia is not enough, under normal circumstances, to cause tissue hypoxia.

IV.26   TTFTT

C   There will be a bounding pulse, which usually indicates a wide pulse pressure.

D   Infection and hypoxia cause confusion.

E   Pursed lips is sometimes described as 'auto-PEEP'. It is a learned manoeuvre to help keep the airways open.

IV.27   FTTTF

A,E   Haemorrhage and septicaemia are complications of surgery, but are not particularly associated with laparoscopic cholecystectomy.

B   Laparoscopic cholecystectomy has, at the time of writing, the reputation of leading to more cut bile ducts than the open operation. In future, with better training, the incidence may decrease – and perhaps surgeons will become less skilled at *open* operations.

C   Tension pneumothorax can occur if insufflating gas passes into the pleural cavity.

D   The cause is uncertain, but right hypochondrial pain can last several months.

IV.28   FTFTF

A   Abdominal pain is usually colicky, not constant.
C   Obstruction produces gaseous distension and a resonant abdomen. Dullness in the flanks is due to fluid (ascites) or blood.
E   Bowel sounds are tinkling. Sounds are absent in paralytic ileus.

IV.29   FFTFF

A   There are not usually prodromal symptoms.
B   Fluid losses are large and must be replaced.
D   About 5% of patients require insulin therapy.
E   Pancreatic pseudocyst is a common complication but does not always need operative intervention.

IV.30   TTFTF

A   An ileal conduit is better than uretero-colic anastomosis.
C   Patients should reduce their salt intake.
E   Pyelonephritis is almost inevitable.

Paper V Questions

V.1 **Agents that may safely be used during anaesthesia in a 2-year-old child who was badly burned 7 days previously include:**
  A thiopentone
  B propofol
  C suxamethonium
  D atracurium
  E ketamine.

V.2 **A diabetic patient takes glibenclamide but is poorly controlled. The following would be safe methods of managing the diabetes during amputation of a toe:**
  A metformin and glibenclamide on the morning of surgery
  B glucose/insulin/potassium infusion from 07:00 on the morning of surgery
  C the patient should be given breakfast and placed first on the morning list
  D a spinal anaesthetic
  E a 10% glucose infusion and subcutaneous insulin with the premedication.

V.3 **The following methods of airway control will prevent contamination of the lungs by regurgitated gastric contents:**
  A a 5.0 mm microlaryngoscopy tube
  B a silver speaking tracheostomy tube
  C a Brain laryngeal mask airway
  D a 5.0 mm oral RAE tube
  E a 7.0 mm spiral armoured endotracheal tube.

V.4 **The following are true of the triad of anaesthesia:**
  A it was described first by Guedel
  B one component is narcosis
  C one component is autonomic reflex suppression
  D one component is muscular relaxation
  E ether provides all three components of the triad.

V.5 **In a patient suffering from sickle-cell trait:**
  A 30–40% of the total haemoglobin is haemoglobin S
  B sickling occurs at a PaO_2 less than 45 mmHg
  C the use of tourniquets is contraindicated
  D preoperative transfusion is indicated if the haemoglobin concentration is less than 10 g/dl
  E the haemoglobin has normal oxygen affinity.

V.6   Late complications of long-term oro-tracheal intubation include:
A   granuloma pyogenicum
B   tracheal stenosis
C   recurrent laryngeal nerve injury
D   bronchopleural fistula
E   dysphonia.

V.7   Cerebral blood flow:
A   is directly related to cardiac output
B   depends on posture
C   is reduced when bleeding reduces the arterial pressure to 75 mmHg systolic
D   is autoregulated between mean pressures of 40 and 180 mmHg
E   is 30% of the cardiac output.

V.8   The following are true of the nerve supply to the pregnant uterus:
A   sensation from the upper segment travels with the sympathetic nerves to T11 and T12
B   sensation from the birth canal is transmitted via the pudendal nerve
C   sensation from the lower segment travels via L2, 3 and 4
D   motor function is served by both sympathetic and parasympathetic nerves
E   an intact nerve supply is essential to initiate the process of normal labour.

V.9   Likely causes of postoperative apnoea in an ex-premature neonate include:
A   hypothermia
B   peroperative opioids
C   residual effects of neuromuscular blockade
D   hypotension
E   hypoglycaemia.

V.10   The ventilatory depressant effects of morphine can be countered by:
A   inhalation of 5% carbon dioxide in oxygen
B   infusion of physostigmine
C   intravenous naltrexone
D   intravenous naloxone
E   infusion of doxapram.

V.11 **The following are causes of high plasma concentrations of serum cholinesterase:**
A   alcoholism
B   ecothiopate therapy
C   pregnancy
D   thyrotoxicosis
E   obesity.

V.12 **The following drugs have the recognised complication of causing postoperative convulsions:**
A   propofol
B   ketamine
C   enflurane
D   doxapram
E   methohexitone.

V.13 **The following are true of the nerve supply to the arm:**
A   the musculocutaneous nerve supplies skin between the mid-upper arm and the lateral epicondyle
B   the lateral cutaneous nerve of forearm supplies skin between the lateral epicondyle and the base of the thumb
C   the hand should be pronated if the arm is abducted in an anaesthetised subject
D   the median nerve passes beneath the flexor retinaculum at the wrist
E   the circumflex nerve is susceptible to injury as it traverses the spiral groove of the humerus.

V.14 **The following are true of the sacrum:**
A   it consists of five fused vertebrae
B   the sacral hiatus represents the absent last neural arch
C   the hiatus is the caudal limit of the extradural space
D   the anatomy is constant between individuals
E   the volume of the adult sacral canal is 20–25 ml.

V.15 **Damage to the facial nerve during a superficial parotidectomy:**
A   can be prevented by avoiding the use of non-depolarising muscle relaxants
B   will result in partial loss of corneal sensation
C   will result in the patient having a lop-sided smile
D   will result in loss of sweating over the affected part
E   will result in partial loss of taste.

V.16   The cervical plexus:

A   is formed by the anterior primary rami
B   receives the ansa hypoglossi from the XIIth cranial nerve
C   supplies cutaneous sensation to the anterior chest wall down to the third rib
D   supplies motor fibres to levator scapulae, sternomastoid and trapezius
E   supplies sensation to the forehead.

V.17   The following are true of coarctation of the aorta:

A   notching is best seen in the first and second ribs
B   girls are more commonly affected than boys
C   there is an association with a bicuspid aortic valve
D   the lesion should be treated conservatively until puberty
E   intraoperative invasive blood pressure is best measured in the left arm.

V.18   There is a slow regular pulse in:

A   complete heart block
B   idioventricular rhythm
C   nodal rhythm
D   a 2:1 atrio-ventricular block
E   constrictive pericarditis.

V.19   There is a fixed low cardiac output:

A   in the neonate
B   in complete heart block
C   in severe aortic stenosis
D   following cardiac transplantation
E   in constrictive pericarditis.

V.20   The following are true of hypoglycaemic coma:

A   the patient is likely to be sweaty
B   the pupils are dilated
C   the pulse volume is good
D   it is a feature of Addison's disease
E   glucagon can be given intramuscularly.

V.21   Splenomegaly occurs in:

A   tuberculosis
B   hereditary spherocytosis
C   porphyria
D   carcinoma of the head of the pancreas
E   thyrotoxicosis.

V.22 Causes of diffuse hepatomegaly include:

A haemochromatosis
B tricuspid incompetence
C constrictive pericarditis
D myelofibrosis
E tuberculosis.

V.23 In a patient with known myasthenia gravis and progressive weakness:

A intravenous neostigmine will produce immediate improvement
B hypokalaemia may be a contributing factor
C all oral medication should be temporarily withdrawn
D thymectomy is indicated
E atropine will produce symptomatic improvement.

V.24 Methaemoglobinaemia is a recognised complication of treatment with:

A sulphonamides
B procaine
C sodium nitroprusside
D phenacetin
E nitrous oxide.

V.25 Features of acute glomerulonephritis include:

A oliguria
B hypertension
C periorbital oedema
D early onset of ascites
E haematuria.

V.26 The development of a spontaneous pneumothorax is associated with:

A congenital lung bullae
B cigarette smoking
C rheumatoid arthritis
D hydatid lung disease
E asthma.

V.27 A 49-year-old man arrives in casualty complaining of epigastric pain that radiates through to the back. He is dyspnoeic, centrally cyanosed and has absent bowel sounds. The following are likely diagnoses:

A acute pancreatitis
B dissecting aortic aneurysm
C myocardial infarction
D perforated duodenal ulcer
E ascending cholangitis.

V.28   Indications for a porta-caval shunt in portal hypertension include:

A   bleeding that is resistant to vasopressin
B   increasing jaundice
C   failure to control bleeding by endoscopic banding
D   failure to halt bleeding after a Sengstaken tube has been in place for 48 h
E   recurring troublesome ascites.

V.29   The following are features of acute appendicitis:

A   pain that is initially poorly localised
B   persistent vomiting
C   early development of pyrexia
D   a leucocytosis of 10 000 cells/mm^3
E   perforation is more likely in patients less than 2 years old.

V.30   The following are true of a supracondylar fracture of the humerus:

A   it is an injury that tends to occur in children
B   nerve damage is uncommon
C   closed reduction is usually satisfactory
D   loss of the radial pulse is an indication for urgent surgery
E   Volkmann's ischaemic contracture is a complication.

Paper V Answers

V.1 **TFFTT**

B At the time of writing, the data sheet for propofol states that it should not be used for induction of anaesthesia in children under 3 years old.

C Suxamethonium can cause hyperkalaemia after severe burns. The quoted danger period is usually in the order of weeks after the event, but suxamethonium is probably better avoided.

V.2 **FTFTT**

These branches are not mutually exclusive. There are several safe ways of giving this anaesthetic.

A Combination therapy can be used postoperatively but is not safe during operation.

C This method is dangerous.

B,D, Not everyone would agree, but done correctly these
E options are safe.

V.3 **TFFFT**

A,E The microlaryngoscopy and armoured tubes are cuffed. The speaking tube and the RAE tube are not.

C The laryngeal mask airway does not protect against regurgitation and aspiration.

V.4 **FTFTT**

A The triad was described in 1950 by Rees and Gray. Questions on history may not be asked in the MCQ examination, but will certainly be asked in the vivas. History also provides a good way to start essays. As with all other subjects, you cannot (and are not expected) to know everything.

B–D You can argue that we use the autonomic reflexes to judge analgesia perioperatively, but the triad of anaesthesia is clearly defined by the three properties: narcosis, analgesia and relaxation.

V.5 **TTTFT**

D Transfusion is rarely indicated by a haemoglobin concentration of 10 g/dl, whether or not the patient has sickle-cell trait.

E Haemoglobin S has normal oxygen affinity, but is less soluble than normal haemoglobin.

V.6   TTTFT

C   There are case reports of damage to the recurrent laryngeal nerve and the lingual nerve.

D   Bronchopleural fistula is not a documented complication of orotracheal intubation.

V.7   FFTFF

A   In heavy exercise, cardiac output increases fivefold because of blood flow to muscle. Cerebral blood flow is not affected.

C,D   Autoregulation applies between mean arterial pressures of 60 and 140 mmHg. (The existence of autoregulation is another reason why **A** cannot be 'true'.)

E   Cerebral blood flow is 15% of cardiac output.

V.8   TTFTF

C   Sensation from the lower segment travels via the sacral parasympathetics: S2–4.

E   Normal labour occurs in patients with transection of the spinal cord.

V.9   TTTFT

B   Ex-premature babies are more sensitive to the effects of opioids than term babies.

D   Hypotension would have to be very severe and therefore is not a likely cause.

V.10   TFFTT

The question says 'countered' not 'reversed'.

A   Opioids shift the carbon dioxide response curve to the right, so patients' ventilation is less at any given carbon dioxide tension. But carbon dioxide still stimulates the breathing.

B   Physostigmine is an anticholinesterase that crosses the blood–brain barrier, but it does not counter the effects of opioids.

C   Naltrexone is an oral opioid antagonist used in the maintenance therapy of drug addicts. It cannot be used with opioid agonists.

V.11 TFFTT

B   Ecothiopate is a cholinesterase inhibitor. It can reduce the effect (not the concentration) of serum cholinesterase. It certainly does not cause increased concentrations of the enzyme. Ecothiopate is a drug that seems to occur more in anaesthesia examinations than in patients.

C   There are *low* concentrations in pregnancy, especially in the second half of pregnancy.

V.12 TTTTT

The question does not ask about epilepsy, nor does it ask specifically for *epileptiform* convulsions. But all these drugs have the recognised complication of causing postoperative involuntary seizures, which are convulsions whether or not they are truly epileptic.

V.13 FTTTF

A,B   The musculocutaneous nerve terminates as the lateral cutaneous nerve of forearm.

E   The radial nerve traverses the spiral groove. The circumflex can be damaged as it runs round the surgical neck of the humerus.

V.14 TTTFT

C   The sacral hiatus is roofed by the posterior sacro-coccygeal ligaments.

D   The anatomy is notoriously variable, which is a great nuisance to anaesthetists.

V.15 FFTFF

A   The use of relaxants has no influence of itself, but avoidance of muscle relaxation (or allowing partial reversal) enables the surgeon to use a nerve stimulator to identify the branches of the nerve.

B,D   Corneal sensation and sweating are trigeminal.

E   The damage is too distal to affect taste.

V.16 TFTTF

B The hypoglossal (XII) *forms* the ansa hypoglossi *with* contributions from C1–3.

D The cervical plexus does supply sternomastoid and trapezius, but their main supply is from the spinal accessory nerve (XI).

E The face is supplied by the trigeminal nerve (V).

V.17 FFTFF

A The notching of coarctation is best seen in lower ribs.

B Males are affected more commonly.

D Coarctation is best treated earlier, before hypertension develops. *Diagnosis* is often delayed.

E The left subclavian is often clamped during resection and the right arm is therefore preferred for invasive monitoring.

V.18 TTTTF

E There will be a sinus tachycardia in constrictive pericarditis.

V.19 FFTFT

A Stroke volume varies little, but rate alters.

B Rate is fixed, but stroke volume varies, though not greatly in elderly patients.

D The transplanted heart is denervated, but it can respond to changes in preload and to endogenous hormones.

V.20 TTTTT

A–C Hypoglycaemia causes signs of sympathetic overactivity.

E Glucagon can be given, although intravenous glucose is the more usual treatment.

V.21 TTTTF

D Pancreatic carcinoma occludes the portal vein.

E Thyrotoxicosis does not cause splenomegaly.

V.22   TFTTT

B   Tricuspid *stenosis* causes liver enlargement because of
         the resulting increased venous pressure.

V.23   FTTFF

A   Neostigmine can make things worse if the patient is in
         cholinergic crisis.
D   Thymectomy is not first-line treatment for progressive
         weakness.
E   Atropine is a muscarinic antagonist.

V.24   TFTTF

B   Prilocaine, not procaine, causes methaemoglobinaemia.
E   Nitrous oxide is unrelated chemically to nitrites. It does
         not cause methaemoglobinaemia.

V.25   TTTFT

B   The hypertension of acute glomerulonephritis is caused
         by many things: increased extracellular fluid volume,
         increased cardiac output and an increased peripheral
         vascular resistance.
C,D   Oedema can develop first periorbitally, but eventually
         becomes generalised.

V.26   TFFTT

B   Cigarette smoking is not a cause of spontaneous
         pneumothorax.
C   Rheumatoid lung does not predispose to spontaneous
         pneumothorax.

V.27   TFFFF

This is a tricky clinical question. Look at all the points, they
must *all* fit. This is a false situation: you never have to make
diagnoses on this type of half-information – but this is what is
often presented in examinations.

A   Cyanosis is a well recognised feature of acute
         pancreatitis, and is due to a combination of circulatory
         collapse and release of vasoactive peptides.
B,E   Cyanosis does not usually occur in patients with
         dissecting aneurysm or perforated duodenal ulcer.
C   Myocardial infarction will cause cyanosis if there is heart
         failure, but epigastric pain radiating through to the back is
         an uncommon presentation of myocardial infarction. Also,
         absent bowel sounds are not a feature of an
         uncomplicated myocardial infarction.

V.28   FFTFF

Vasopressin and Sengstaken tubes are now recommended only as stop gap measures until the patient can be referred to a centre able to coagulate or band the bleeding points.
Porta-caval shunting should be restricted to those patients in whom banding fails.

V.29   TFFTT

B   Vomiting occurs early but is not usually persistent.
C   Pyrexia and tachycardia do not occur early, and the pyrexia is not usually extreme.
E   The risk of perforation, and of death, are both much greater in babies.

V.30   TTTFT

B   The median and ulnar nerves can be damaged, but damage is uncommon.
D   Loss of the radial pulse is an indication for strict observation but surgery is not needed provided that the circulation is adequate.

Paper VI Questions

VI.1 Untreated preoperative hypertension:

A   increases the incidence of perioperative myocardial infarction
B   should be treated before surgery
C   is a contraindication to the use of isoflurane
D   reduces the risk of deep venous thrombosis
E   is a contraindication to intraoperative use of epidural analgesia.

VI.2 In a 7-year-old child undergoing general anaesthesia for elective adeno-tonsillectomy:

A   nasal intubation allows better surgical access
B   a laryngeal mask airway (LMA) is contraindicated
C   intravenous induction is contraindicated
D   throat packs are frequently not used
E   trimeprazine 4 mg/kg is suitable premedication.

VI.3 Factors which increase the likelihood of regurgitation at induction include:

A   obesity
B   anxiety
C   upper respiratory obstruction
D   increased 'barrier' pressure
E   hiccoughs.

VI.4   Recognised causes of postoperative jaundice include:
A   blood transfusion
B   halothane hepatitis
C   infective hepatitis
D   Weil's disease
E   renal failure.

VI.5   A 23-year-old motor cyclist is brought into casualty unconscious. His blood pressure is 80/40 mmHg and his pulse rate is 115. He has no broken limbs and clinically he has a right-sided pneumothorax. The following are true:
A   the most likely cause of the cardiovascular signs is a tension pneumothorax
B   if he is cyanosed, adult respiratory distress syndrome (ARDS) is a possible cause
C   the hypotension is severe enough to account for the unconsciousness
D   the fast pulse indicates that intracranial pressure is not increased
E   urgent laparotomy is indicated.

VI.6   The following are suitable doses in a fit man weighing 80 kg:
A   25 ml 2% lignocaine with adrenaline by caudal injection for haemorrhoidectomy
B   35 ml 0.5% plain bupivacaine into the lumbar epidural space for bilateral inguinal hernia repairs
C   2.5 ml 0.5% hyperbaric bupivacaine intrathecally for transurethral resection of prostate
D   1.0 ml 0.5% plain bupivacaine intrathecally with patient sitting for anal stretch
E   10 ml 0.5% bupivacaine to provide postoperative pain relief by field block after repair of a hernia.

VI.7   During the last trimester of pregnancy:
A   resting $PaCO_2$ is decreased
B   haematocrit is increased
C   blood volume is increased
D   gastric secretion is increased
E   total peripheral resistance is reduced.

VI.8   Symptoms or signs likely to occur in amniotic fluid embolism include:
A   cyanosis
B   hypofibrinogenaemia
C   chest pain
D   hypoventilation
E   hypertension.

VI.9 The following statements about anticholinergic drugs are true:
A glycopyrronium is eliminated from the body more quickly than atropine.
B both atropine and hyoscine increase pulmonary dead space
C atropine premedication is contraindicated in febrile children
D 4.0 mg atropine is required to produce complete vagal blockade in a 70 kg man
E hyoscine is contraindicated in elderly patients.

VI.10 EMLA (eutectic mixture of local anaesthetics) cream:
A contains one part lignocaine to three parts prilocaine
B causes methaemoglobinaemia in small children
C reaches its peak effect at 45 minutes
D is useful topical analgesia after circumcision in a young boy
E anaesthetises the eardrum for insertion of grommets.

VI.11 The following statements about the flammability of anaesthetic gases are true:
A enflurane will not burn at atmospheric pressure
B ethyl chloride spray does not burn
C grease will ignite spontaneously in high pressure oxygen
D ether burns if heated above its boiling point
E extensive internal burns are a recognised risk of using nitrous oxide insufflation during laparoscopy.

VI.12 The following are true of the nose and nasal cavity:
A the medial wall of the nasal cavity is partly cartilaginous
B there are three separate turbinate bones
C the best route for nasal intubation is below the inferior turbinate
D the paranasal sinuses are not fully developed until adolescence
E septoplasty can be performed under topical analgesia.

VI.13   The femoral artery:

A   is the continuation of the external iliac artery
B   is readily palpable throughout its length
C   is separated from the hip joint only by the tendon of psoas major
D   lies medial to the femoral nerve just below the inguinal ligament
E   in some subjects follows an aberrant course known as the profunda femora.

VI.14   The following are true of the oculomotor nerve:

A   it enters the superior orbital fissure via the cavernous sinus
B   it supplies sympathetic and parasympathetic innervation to the eye
C   fibres subserving reflex activity synapse in the superior colliculus
D   a palsy results in a relaxed pupil, fixed at mid-dilatation
E   a palsy results in a convergent squint.

VI.15   The medial popliteal (tibial) nerve:

A   is the larger of the two terminal branches of the sciatic nerve
B   supplies the muscles of the calf
C   gives an articular division to the knee
D   subserves sensation over the posterolateral aspect of lower leg and foot
E   terminates by dividing into the medial and lateral plantar nerves.

VI.16   Clinical findings consistent with persistent vomiting for 4 days include:

A   vitamin B_{12} deficiency anaemia
B   a blood urea of 12 mmol/l
C   hypokalaemia
D   hypochloraemia
E   tetany.

VI.17   Causes of syncope include:

A   diabetes
B   aortic incompetence
C   hypertrophic obstructive cardiomyopathy
D   coughing
E   hypercapnia.

VI.18 Suitable treatment for paroxysmal atrial tachycardia includes:
A   beta-adrenergic blockade
B   anticholinesterase therapy
C   carotid sinus massage
D   adenosine
E   intravenous lignocaine.

VI.19 In the Wolff–Parkinson–White syndrome:
A   there is a short PR interval on the ECG
B   heart failure is not a recognised feature
C   amiodarone is an effective long-term treatment
D   the patient can terminate the attacks by manoeuvres that increase vagal tone
E   a cardiac pacemaker is the preferred operative treatment.

VI.20 Indications for ventilation in a patient with Guillain–Barré syndrome include:
A   forced vital capacity (FVC) less than 15 ml/kg
B   total lung capacity less than 3 litres
C $PaCO_2$ above 7 kPa (52 mmHg)
D   loss of laryngeal reflexes
E   proximal neuropathy in all four limbs.

VI.21 The following are true of ulcerative colitis:
A   sarcomas develop in the large bowel
B   medical treatment includes immunosuppression and steroids
C   colectomy should include excision of the rectum
D   it is associated with hepatic dysfunction
E   it is usually a self-limiting condition.

VI.22 A haemoglobin of 8 g/dl with a reticulocyte count of 10% occurs in:
A   aplastic anaemia
B   untreated pernicious anaemia
C   polycythaemia
D   haemolytic anaemia
E   acute leukaemia.

VI.23 Polyneuropathy is a recognised feature of:
A   myasthenia gravis
B   mercury poisoning
C   alcoholism
D   polyarteritis nodosa
E   bronchogenic carcinoma.

VI.24   Perioperative oliguria occurs because of:

A   antidiuretic hormone release
B   stimulation of aldosterone release
C   the third space effect
D   a specific effect of anaesthesia on renal tubules
E   hyperglycaemia.

VI.25   A reduction in the diffusing capacity of the lung occurs in:

A   emphysema
B   polycythaemia
C   pulmonary embolism
D   Hamman–Rich syndrome
E   laparoscopic surgery.

VI.26   Blood for gas analysis is taken from a 63-year-old man with an acute exacerbation of chronic bronchitis. The following results are compatible with this diagnosis:

A PaO_2 5.6 kPa (42 mmHg)
B $PaCO_2$ 10.4 kPa (78 mmHg)
C   pH 7.58
D   standard base excess 8.3 mmol/l
E   standard bicarbonate 18 mmol/l.

VI.27   Hormone manipulation is a treatment for patients with advanced breast carcinoma. Those likely to respond include those:

A   who are more than 5 years past the menopause at first presentation
B   whose metastases are primarily in soft tissue
C   with advanced local disease only
D   with a short interval free from recurrence
E   with tumours positive for oestrogen receptors.

VI.28   Shortly after perforation of a duodenal ulcer:

A   the axillary temperature is subnormal
B   there is maximum tenderness in the right iliac fossa
C   there is shoulder pain
D   serum amylase is increased
E   there is haemodilution.

VI.29 **A 5-year-old child is suspected of having acute appendicitis.**
   The following are likely to confirm this diagnosis:
   A   a rectal temperature of 40°C
   B   bronchial breathing at the right lung base
   C   a urinary sample with 5 white cells per high-power field
   D   pain in the right iliac fossa when pressing on the left of the abdomen
   E   diarrhoea the previous evening.

VI.30 **In benign prostatic hypertrophy:**
   A   patients have to strain to start their stream
   B   frequency is the earliest symptom
   C   chronic retention should not be decompressed rapidly
   D   an excretory pyelogram should be obtained if there is renal failure
   E   an episode of acute retention is an indication for elective prostatectomy.

Paper VI Answers

VI.1 FTFFF

The blood pressure at which an elective procedure should be postponed is a good topic for discussion. For this question, you can assume the hypertension is severe enough to require treatment.

A The incidence of perioperative infarction is increased only if there is a recent history of myocardial infarction, or, more controversially, if there is marked coronary artery disease.

B At your final exam, you should be able to discuss hypertension, anaesthesia and surgery intelligently: you may even disagree with our answer, but you must be able to give reasons for your decision.

C Isoflurane may stabilise the blood pressure during the procedure, but hypertension can recur postoperatively.

D There is no association between hypertension and the risk of deep venous thrombosis.

E There is no reason not to use an epidural, either during or after the operation. The usual precautions would have to be taken – and perhaps special care to avoid sudden decreases in blood pressure.

VI.2 FFFTF

A Young children are not usually intubated nasally, and a nasal tube is *less* convenient for adenoidectomy.

B Flexible wire reinforced LMAs can be used for intraoral surgery.

C Questions on the bleeding tonsil are stock questions in anaesthesia examinations (and there are MCQs in this book on the subject). But there is no contraindication to intravenous induction in an elective case. It is very easy in the examination room to misinterpret questions: this question is not about emergency anaesthesia.

E The maximum dose recommended for trimeprazine in the data sheet is now 2 mg/kg.

VI.3 TTTFT

D Regurgitation is *less* likely if the barrier pressure of the lower oesophageal sphincter is increased.

E Reflux of gastric contents is almost inevitable if the patient hiccoughs. Regurgitation is much less likely, but hiccoughs increase the overall likelihood.

VI.4   TTTFF

A,C   Blood transfusion can cause jaundice if there is haemolysis, or through transmission of infections such as non-A, non-B hepatitis.

B   Halothane hepatitis is rare, but is definitely a recognised cause of jaundice after an operation.

D   Weil's disease is a spirochaetal infection. Any association with operations would be coincidental.

E   Renal failure can be a consequence of liver failure, but is not a cause of jaundice.

VI.5   FFFFF

All these answers have a grain of truth in them, but they are all false.

A   The most likely cause of the cardiovascular signs is bleeding: into the abdomen or the thorax, or from the head.

B   It is too early for ARDS. Cyanosis at this stage is likely to be due to tension pneumothorax, aspiration or central respiratory depression because of a head injury.

C   A systolic pressure of 80 mmHg in a previously fit young man will not cause unconsciousness.

D   A slow pulse is not inevitable when intracranial pressure is increased.

E   There is urgent need for laparotomy only if abdominal trauma is suspected.

VI.6   TTTFF

There is no absolute 'correct dose'; the volume necessary will vary from patient to patient. Having said that:

D   Plain bupivacaine is isobaric or slightly hypobaric. The block produced by 1 ml is likely to be unpredictable: heavy bupivacaine is better.

E   A larger volume than 10 ml is needed for good postoperative pain relief.

VI.7   TFTFT

B   Haematocrit decreases in the third trimester.

D   Gastric secretion does not alter, but gastric emptying is delayed.

VI.8   TTTFF

D   In amniotic fluid embolism, acute hypoxia causes hyperventilation.

E   There is hypotension caused by peripheral vasodilation and myocardial depression.

VI.9   TTTFT

A   The elimination half-life of glycopyrronium is less than an hour, and that of atropine is 2.5 h.

B   Bronchodilation increases bronchiolar volume and hence anatomical dead space.

D   The vagus is blocked by 2–3 mg atropine.

E   Hyoscine causes confusion in the elderly.

VI.10   FTFFF

A   EMLA is 25 mg lignocaine and 2 mg prilocaine per gram.

B   Methaemoglobinaemia has been reported following its repeated use in small children for blood sampling.

C   EMLA must be left for at least 1 hour, except before treatment of genital warts, when peak effect is at 15 minutes.

D   EMLA is formulated in high concentration to pass intact skin, but the genital skin is thin. High plasma concentrations occur if it is applied to broken skin or to the genital region. EMLA can cause methaemoglobinaemia and is contraindicated.

E   EMLA is potentially ototoxic and should not be used for procedures that might allow it to penetrate to the middle ear.

VI.11   TFTFT

Most operating theatres are still 'anti-static' even though the risk of explosions has been largely eliminated by the withdrawal of ether and cyclopropane from anaesthesia in the UK.

B   Spray ampoules of ethyl chloride are still available. They are used for (not very effective) cryoanalgesia and to test sensory levels after regional blockade. Ethyl chloride is a potent general anaesthetic, though not used nowadays for general anaesthesia. It is flammable and explosive when mixed with oxygen.

C   Grease must not be applied to oxygen or nitrous oxide pipelines.

D   The boiling point of ether is 36°C at one atmosphere pressure, but this is irrelevant to when it is able to burn once first ignited.

E   Nitrous oxide does not burn, but will support combustion.

VI.12   TFTTF

B   Only the inferior turbinate is a separate bone, the upper and middle turbinates are part of the ethmoid.

E   The base of the septum and the columella need the injection of some local anaesthetic because they are covered by squamous epithelium not by mucous membrane.

VI.13 TFTTF

C An important point of applied anatomy: it is easy, especially in infants, to puncture the hip joint when attempting a femoral stab.

E The profunda femora is a large vessel that is the main blood supply to the adductors, flexors and extensors of the thigh.

VI.14 TFTFF

B,D The oculomotor nerve supplies parasympathetic fibres. An oculomotor palsy causes a dilated pupil because of unopposed sympathetic action.

E A palsy causes a *divergent* squint: the muscles *not* supplied are the lateral rectus and superior oblique.

VI.15 TTTTT

D There is a variable contribution from the lateral popliteal.

E The plantar nerves supply the sole of the foot, and the lateral plantar (equivalent to the ulnar in the hand) supplies most of the small muscles of the foot.

VI.16 FTTTT

A Vitamin B_{12} deficiency takes several months to develop.

B The blood urea is increased because of dehydration.

VI.17 TFTTF

A There is autonomic neuropathy in diabetes.

B Aortic stenosis, not incompetence, causes syncope.

E Syncope occurs when hypocapnia is caused by hysterical (or intentional) hyperventilation.

VI.18   TFTTF

    B   Anticholinesterases cause bradycardia but are not used to treat tachycardias.

    E   Lignocaine is not effective in supraventricular dysrhythmias.

VI.19   TFTTF

    B   Failure of output occurs in extreme tachycardia.

    D   Sometimes techniques such as the Valsalva manoeuvre can terminate an attack.

    E   Ablation of the aberrant pathway by open surgery or via a catheter is preferred to over-ride pacing.

VI.20   TFTTF

    B   Total lung capacity is not affected by Guillain–Barré syndrome.

    C   The disease can progress rapidly and signs of respiratory failure must be treated properly and promptly. A $PaCO_2$ above 7 kPa indicates severe ventilatory difficulties.

    E   Proximal neuropathy is characteristic, but not an indication for ventilation.

VI.21   FTTTF

    A   Adenocarcinomas develop in the colon and rectum, hence **C**.

    E   Ulcerative colitis is usually a relapsing condition.

VI.22   FFFTF

    The reticulocyte count is a measure of bone marrow response. Disease of the bone marrow reduces the response, hence the only 'true' branch is **D**.

VI.23   FTTTT

    A   Myasthenia gravis affects only the neuromuscular junction.

    C   Polyneuropathy occurs in alcoholism because of the chronic alcohol intake and also because of associated malnutrition.

    D   Polyneuropathy occurs in 70% of patients with the rare condition of polyarteritis nodosa.

    E   Lung cancer has many non-metastatic systemic manifestations and is a very common disease.

VI.24   **TFTFF**

B   Aldosterone does not have a clinically measurable effect on perioperative urine output.

D   The only direct nephrotoxic effect of anaesthesia was the polyuric renal failure caused by methoxyflurane, which is obsolete.

E   Glucose is an osmotic diuretic.

VI.25   **TFTTF**

D   Hamman–Rich syndrome is a fibrosing alveolitis. Do not worry about not recognising eponyms of unusual diseases.

E   A pneumoperitoneum does not alter diffusing capacity, though it may change functional residual capacity.

VI.26   **TTFTF**

Not all patients with chronic bronchitis retain carbon dioxide. If they do, between acute attacks they will be mildly acidotic, an increased bicarbonate partly compensating for the increased carbon dioxide.

C   Whether or not the patient is a retainer, an acute attack will make him acidotic.

D,E   If he is a retainer, then he will 'normally' have a base excess. If he is not a retainer, he will not have a base excess – but there is no reason (from the information given) for him to have a metabolic acidosis (**E**). If he remains ill, a metabolic acidosis may develop (secondary to serious infection, heart failure, or whatever) and complicate his acid-base status, but this question is about an 'acute' exacerbation.

VI.27   **TFTFT**

B,D   Patients with more aggressive disease and with metastases are less likely to do well. This is not a universal rule for all cancers. Chemotherapy is often more effective (at least initially) in more aggressive disease.

VI.28   **TFTFF**

A   A subnormal temperature is apparently a feature of early perforation (at least in the surgical textbooks).

B   Abdominal pain is likely to be central.

C   Air under the diaphragm causes shoulder tip pain.

D   Serum amylase is used to differentiate from acute pancreatitis.

E   There is no reason for haemodilution. The patient is likely to develop haemoconcentration later unless adequately resuscitated.

VI.29   TFFTF

The important words are 'symptoms *likely to confirm* the diagnosis'.

B,C, All these would, if anything, make the diagnosis doubtful.

E

VI.30   FTTFF

A   Straining is no help: the patient must just wait.

D   An intravenous pyelogram is performed *unless* there is renal failure.

E   At the time of writing, the reason this branch is 'false' is that urine flow studies must be done before elective prostatectomy is considered. There are many other treatments for benign prostatic hypertrophy under investigation, and a different reason will probably be the correct one in a few years' time.

Paper VII Questions

VII.1 **Features of rheumatoid arthritis that may influence anaesthetic management when there is coincidental surgery include:**
A stridor
B amyloidosis of the kidney
C pulmonary fibrosis
D erosion of the odontoid peg
E polycythaemia.

VII.2 **During cardiopulmonary resuscitation:**
A the initial treatment for asystole is defibrillation
B electromechanical dissociation should be treated by 1 ml of 1:10 000 adrenaline intravenously
C the initial DC shock in an adult is 200 J
D the first choice drug for pulseless ventricular tachycardia is lignocaine 100 mg intravenously
E atropine 3 mg intravenously may be beneficial in electromechanical dissociation.

VII.3 **Concerning gases and cylinders:**
A working pressure of a modern anaesthetic machine is 60 lb/in² (4 bar)
B the filling ratio of a nitrous oxide cylinder is 0.75
C blue cylinders with white 'shoulders' contain liquid nitrous oxide at room temperature
D the pressure inside a full oxygen cylinder is about 2000 lb/in² (132 bar)
E a cylinder of carbon dioxide does not require a reducing valve.

VII.4 **Opioid premedication:**
A reduces total perioperative opioid requirements
B can be given orally
C is contraindicated in children
D slows gastric emptying
E promotes hepatic clearance of anaesthetic agents.

VII.5   Decompression sickness:
A   causes avascular necrosis of bone
B   is due to an alveolar oxygen deficit
C   is cured by breathing a mixture of oxygen and helium
D   occurs up to 24 h after the decompression
E   is avoided if helium is included in the inspired gas mixture.

VII.6   Characteristic direct features of overdosage of a tricyclic antidepressant include:
A   convulsions
B   metabolic acidosis
C   cardiac arrhythmias
D   hypothermia
E   respiratory alkalosis.

VII.7   Intracranial pressure is reduced by:
A   intravenous mannitol
B   halothane
C   phenytoin
D   barbiturates
E   suxamethonium.

VII.8   Acute inversion of the uterus following delivery causes:
A   cyanosis
B   hypotension
C   bradycardia
D   hypofibrinogenaemia
E   severe haemorrhage.

VII.9   A 6-month-old infant of Greek parents presents with a 1-week history of malaise and anorexia. There are multiple bruises on the limbs and scalp, inflamed and swollen gums, a rectal temperature of 38°C, and a painful left leg held in flexion. Likely diagnoses include:
A   scurvy
B   septicaemia secondary to osteomyelitis
C   haemophilia
D   child abuse
E   idiopathic thrombocytopenia.

VII.10 **Intraoperative analgesia in man is satisfactorily achieved with:**
A phenoperidine
B clonidine
C etorphine
D ketamine
E indoramin.

VII.11 **Suxamethonium will cause clinically important increases in serum potassium concentration in patients suffering from:**
A pseudohypertrophic muscular dystrophy
B uraemia
C tetanus
D paraplegia
E diabetes mellitus.

VII.12 **When a pleural drain is inserted for pneumothorax:**
A subcutaneous tissues down to the pleura should be blunt dissected
B the drain must be held firmly to prevent the trocar point being pushed back during insertion
C the drain should be connected to the underwater tube of the sealing valve
D the underwater seal container should be able to hold a large volume of fluid
E if suction is required a low-volume high-suction pump is required.

VII.13 **The following complications may follow unilateral supraclavicular block of the brachial plexus:**
A respiratory paralysis
B puncture of the subclavian artery
C pneumothorax
D dural puncture
E epileptiform convulsions.

VII.14 **The extradural space:**
A is connected to the pleural cavity
B extends from the fourth ventricle to the sacral hiatus
C contains fat, arteries and veins but no lymphatic vessels
D has valveless veins that provide a direct connection between the pelvic and cerebral veins
E provides a recirculation pathway for extravasated cerebrospinal fluid.

VII.15 **The following are true of the facial nerve:**
A it supplies salivary secretomotor fibres
B it supplies lacrimal secretomotor fibres
C an intracranial lesion usually involves the auditory nerve as well
D compression by an acoustic neuroma will not cause paralysis of the forehead
E it traverses the eardrum.

VII.16 **An increased plasma bicarbonate occurs in:**
A renal failure
B persistent vomiting
C diabetes insipidus
D rheumatoid arthritis
E hepatic coma.

VII.17 **Suitable methods for the treatment of paroxysmal atrial tachycardia include:**
A carotid sinus massage
B disopyramide
C synchronised DC defibrillation
D amiodarone
E adenosine.

VII.18 **Digoxin has the following effects on the electrocardiogram:**
A increased R–R interval
B shortened Q–T interval
C first degree heart block
D prominent U waves
E effects proportional to the efficacy of treatment.

VII.19 **A low, fixed cardiac output occurs in:**
A aortic stenosis
B constrictive pericarditis
C mitral stenosis
D cor pulmonale
E digoxin toxicity.

VII.20 **The following are true of carcinoid syndrome:**
A the primary is commonly in the appendix
B it occurs only if there are secondaries in the liver
C the patient is usually constipated
D asthmatic attacks occur
E tricuspid stenosis is a rare complication.

VII.21 Complications of rheumatoid arthritis include:

A anaemia
B pericarditis
C peripheral arteritis
D jaundice
E splenomegaly.

VII.22 Chronic diarrhoea is associated with:

A a Meckel's diverticulum
B giardiasis
C surgical truncal vagotomy
D diabetic autonomic neuropathy
E viral gastroenteritis.

VII.23 Dystrophia myotonica is associated with:

A thyroid adenoma
B the development of diabetes mellitus
C wasting of the sternomastoid muscles
D a high arched palate
E frontal baldness.

VII.24 Drugs known to increase barrier pressure at the gastro-oesophageal junction include:

A prochlorperazine
B atropine
C glycopyrronium
D fentanyl
E suxamethonium.

VII.25 The following are true of acute pyelonephritis:

A the most common organism is *Strep. faecalis*
B the onset is usually sudden
C it is more common in women
D antibiotic treatment is continued until the urine is sterile
E fluids should be restricted initially to rest the kidneys.

VII.26 Likely causes of a large anterior mediastinal mass seen on a routine chest radiograph include:

A thymic cyst
B lymphoma
C unfolded aorta
D retrosternal goitre
E diaphragmatic hernia.

VII.27   Abdominal pain is a prominent feature of:
A   staphylococcal food poisoning
B   typhoid fever
C   paralytic ileus
D   lead poisoning
E   Crohn's disease.

VII.28   Likely complications of abdominoperineal resection of the rectum include:
A   deep venous thrombosis
B   paralytic ileus
C   air embolism
D   postoperative atelectasis
E   uraemia.

VII.29   Acute peptic ulceration:
A   is common after ingestion of aspirin
B   is frequently multiple
C   usually causes perforation
D   sometimes occurs in the duodenum soon after severe burns
E   generally responds to appropriate antibiotic treatment.

VII.30   The following are true of osteoarthritis of the hip:
A   the condition is virtually unknown in patients below 17 years of age
B   it is commoner in people who take regular exercise
C   it is a self-limiting condition
D   an uncemented prosthesis is recommended in elderly patients
E   late sepsis is an uncommon complication of arthroplasty.

Paper VII Answers

VII.1 TTTTF

E   Anaemia, not polycythaemia, occurs in rheumatoid arthritis.

VII.2 FFTFF

These answers are based upon the 1992 guidelines.

A   A precordial thump is the first line of treatment after initial basic resuscitation.

B   The dose is 1 mg, which is 1 ml of 1:1000.

D   The first choice drug in pulseless ventricular tachycardia is adrenaline.

E   Atropine is recommended in asystole, but not in electromechanical dissociation.

VII.3 TTFTF

B   The filling ratio is the proportion of the cylinder initially filled with liquid nitrous oxide. The ratio is less in cylinders used in the tropics.

C   Blue and white cylinders contain Entonox, which is in the gaseous phase at room temperature.

E   Carbon dioxide is stored at high pressure and a reducing valve is needed; in cyclopropane cylinders the pressure was only 4 bar.

VII.4 FTFTF

A   This is the idea of pre-emptive analgesia. There is support from theory and animal work but, as yet, no real support from clinical studies.

B   Opioids are not usually given orally preoperatively, but they can be.

C   Doses must be calculated carefully and prescribed explicitly.

E   There is no evidence for this.

VII.5   TFFTF

B   Decompression sickness is caused by bubbles of gas forming in the blood stream. It is nothing to do with hypoxia.

C   It is treated by rapid recompression, usually with high concentrations of oxygen, which assists diffusion of excess nitrogen from the tissues.

D   The onset of the condition may be delayed, especially if the diver then travels by aeroplane.

E   Helium/oxygen mixtures diffuse more quickly from the tissues than air, but decompression sickness can still occur on rapid decompression.

VII.6   TFTFF

B,E   Ventilatory depression causes a respiratory acidosis, but the drugs do not themselves cause a metabolic disturbance.

D   Hyperpyrexia may occur.

VII.7   TFFTF

B   Halothane raises intracranial pressure by causing cerebral vasodilation.

C   Phenytoin has no direct effect. It will lower intracranial pressure if the increase is secondary to epileptic fitting for which the drug was given.

E   Suxamethonium is in all the lists of causes of raised intracranial pressure – but the effect may not be great and is of doubtful importance. Suxamethonium does not *reduce* intracranial pressure.

VII.8   FTFFF

A   There is no impairment of gas exchange.

C   There will be tachycardia.

D,E   Neither are specific associations of inverted uterus.

VII.9   FTFFF

Any diagnosis must fit all the (limited) information you are given. The history, temperature, leg held in flexion and pattern of bleeding suggest only **B** is likely.

VII.10   TFFTF

    B   Clonidine has been investigated as an adjunct to anaesthesia. It may reduce the need for opioids and prolong the action of local anaesthetics, but it is not an analgesic by itself.

    C   Etorphine is an opioid licensed for animal use only.

    E   Indoramin is an alpha$_1$-adrenergic blocker used in the treatment of hypertension: if you don't recognise a drug, leave the answer blank!

VII.11   TTTTF

    D   The answer must be 'true' if no time interval is specified. It takes days to weeks for the sensitivity to occur.

    E   If there is some obscure association it is not common!

VII.12   TFTTF

    B   Modern teaching suggests that the trocar be withdrawn from the tip of the drain tube before insertion to lessen the risk of damaging the lung.

    E   A high-volume low-suction pump is required to prevent air accumulating in the pleural cavity.

VII.13   FTTFT

    A   Unilateral phrenic block is a complication of the supraclavicular approach but even bilateral phrenic blockade does not, in itself, cause respiratory paralysis.

    D   Dural puncture is a complication of the interscalene, not supraclavicular, technique.

    E   Convulsions are a risk of an overdose of local anaesthetic by any route.

VII.14   FFFTF

    A   The thoracic epidural space is separated from the pleural cavity only by the parietal pleura, but there is no direct connection.

    B   The superior boundary is the foramen magnum.

    E   There is not normally cerebrospinal fluid outside the dura.

VII.15   TTTTF

    B   Lacrimal secretomotor fibres travel in the greater
          superficial petrosal nerve.

    D   There is bilateral innervation of the upper facial muscles.

    E   The facial nerve traverses the internal auditory meatus. A
          branch, the chorda tympani, traverses the eardrum.

VII.16   FTFFF

Increased bicarbonate is a primary alkalosis, or compensation
for a respiratory acidosis.

    A   Inability to synthesise bicarbonate in renal failure causes
          metabolic acidosis.

    C,E   There is hypovolaemia in diabetes insipidus but not
           alterations of bicarbonate. Hepatic coma produces a
           metabolic acidosis.

VII.17   TTFTF

    C   Defibrillation is not used for paroxysmal *atrial*
          tachycardia.

    E   Adenosine is suitable for converting supraventricular
          tachycardias, including Wolff–Parkinson–White
          tachycardias, to sinus rhythm. By slowing conduction at
          the A-V node adenosine is useful in the
          electrocardiographic diagnosis of other atrial
          tachycardias, but it is not treatment because of its short
          half-life.

VII.18   TTTFF

    A   Increased R–R interval just means a reduced heart rate. **A**
          and **B** indicate that the patient is taking digoxin; **C**
          indicates overdose; **E**, unfortunately, is not true.

    D   U waves are a variant of normal.

VII.19   TTTFF

    A–C   Stenotic or constrictive lesions produce a fixed output
           state.

    D,E   Low output occurs in cor pulmonale and digoxin toxicity,
           but the output is not fixed.

VII.20   TTFTT

    B   The syndrome requires hepatic secondaries. The primary
          is usually quite small and the liver can metabolise any
          active substances released from it.

    C   Diarrhoea is common.

VII.21   TTTFT

E   Felty's syndrome is splenomegaly, rheumatoid arthritis and leucopenia.

VII.22   FTTTF

C   This once popular operation has become rare as other forms of treatment for peptic ulceration have developed.
E   Viral gastroenteritis causes *acute* diarrhoea.

VII.23   TTTFT

B   Diabetes mellitus is one of several associated endocrine abnormalities.
D   A high arched palate is a feature of Marfan's syndrome.

VII.24   TFFFT

B–D   Anticholinergic drugs and opioids reduce the tone of the lower oesophageal sphincter and therefore reduce barrier pressure. Note that this is a *physiological* description, which does not mean that the incidence of reflux is increased: only *clinical* observations could show whether that is so.

VII.25   FTTFF

A   *E. coli* is the commonest organism in acute pyelonephritis.
D   Urine is *normally* sterile. Antibiotic treatment is continued for longer than this.
E   The patient ought to drink a lot.

VII.26   TTFTF

C,E   Neither an unfolded aorta nor a diaphragmatic hernia give an anterior mediastinal mass.

VII.27   **FFFTT**

A   Staphylococcal food poisoning is more likely to produce just vomiting.

B   Pain is not a feature of typhoid.

C   There may well be concurrent abdominal pain (e.g. postoperative ileus) but the pain is not a feature of the ileus.

D   Colicky pain is present in the alimentary type of lead poisoning.

E   Pain may be masked by the bowel disturbances.

VII.28   **TTFTF**

C,E   There is no particular reason why an abdominoperineal resection should cause air embolism or uraemia, though a careless (or unlucky) surgeon could damage both ureters.

VII.29   **TTFFT**

C   Few peptic ulcers are diagnosed, let alone perforate.

D   It is multiple *stomach* ulcers that can occur after severe burns, though duodenal ulcers may occur later during recovery.

E   Treatment to eliminate *Helicobacter pylori* cures the ulcer in over 80% of cases. Suitable antibiotics are given with antacid. No one regimen is universally accepted at the time of writing.

VII.30   **FFFFT**

A   Osteoarthritis of the hip can occur in the younger age groups following injury or disease (e.g. Perthes disease or a slipped femoral epiphysis).

B   Sports injuries may lead to later osteoarthritis, but regular moderate exercise may protect against the development of arthritis.

C   It is a degenerative 'wear-and-tear' condition that will continue to worsen.

D   Avoiding cement reduces the risk of hypotension, which is probably more dangerous to the elderly. But uncemented prostheses are recommended for *younger* patients, who may need later replacement of the prosthesis.

Paper VIII   Questions

VIII.1 A hypertensive man is controlled on a thiazide diuretic and atenolol (100 mg daily). He presents for anaesthesia for major gastric surgery. He should:

A have his beta-blocker replaced by a calcium channel blocker preoperatively

B have a preoperative electrocardiogram

C continue to receive his antihypertensive therapy up to the time of operation

D receive intravenous beta-blocker during surgery

E only receive 5 ml/kg/h crystalloid replacement to avoid fluid overload.

VIII.2 In a patient presenting with advanced laryngeal carcinoma for elective laryngectomy:

A stridor is uncommon

B intubation should be performed on an anaesthetised patient to avoid the risk of laryngospasm

C antisialogue premedication is desirable

D hypotension and cardiac arrhythmias occur during mobilisation of the larynx

E postoperative disturbances of calcium metabolism are a recognised complication.

VIII.3 Malignant hyperpyrexia:

A develops intraoperatively without any prodromal symptoms or signs

B is precipitated by suxamethonium

C requires monitoring of body temperature for the diagnosis

D is commonly associated with coloured urine

E should be treated initially with intravenous dantrolene 1 g/kg.

VIII.4 The use of nitrous oxide is contraindicated in anaesthesia for:

A severe tracheal stenosis

B resection of the large bowel

C broncho-pleural fistula

D posterior fossa surgery

E cystic pulmonary disease.

VIII.5   Likely complications of infraclavicular subclavian venous cannulation include:

A   recurrent laryngeal nerve palsy
B   air embolism
C   pneumothorax
D   phrenic nerve palsy
E   haemopericardium.

VIII.6   Postoperative cerebral vasospasm occurring in a patient with a subarachnoid haemorrhage:

A   is safe provided that the aneurysm has been clipped successfully
B   may respond to a calcium-channel blocker
C   increases the risk of a subsequent haemorrhage
D   is an absolute indication for postoperative ventilation
E   presents as a hemiplegia.

VIII.7   Satisfactory pre-anaesthetic antacid therapy for caesarean section includes:

A   sodium citrate
B   glycopyrronium
C   metoclopramide
D   ranitidine
E   omeprazole.

VIII.8   Symptoms and signs in a woman with a ruptured ectopic pregnancy and an intra-abdominal blood loss of 1500 ml include:

A   loin discoloration (Grey Turner's sign)
B   hypotension
C   bradycardia
D   shoulder tip pain
E   sweating.

VIII.9   Skin blood flow is:

A   increased by halothane anaesthesia
B   increased in sympathetic activity
C   increased by a lumbar epidural block
D   decreased in barbiturate anaesthesia
E   unchanged in cardiogenic shock.

VIII.10   Drugs which can safely be used in a patient with acute intermittent porphyria include:

A   pethidine
B   chlorpromazine
C   phenylbutazone
D   methohexitone
E   phenytoin.

VIII.11   **A patient presenting for elective abdominal surgery gives a history of chronic obstructive airways disease and is dyspnoeic at rest. Useful tests to establish his fitness for anaesthesia include:**
   A   arterial blood gases
   B   nitrogen washout
   C   ventilatory response to breathing 100% oxygen
   D   spirometry (FEV$_1$ and FVC)
   E   carbon monoxide transfer factor.

VIII.12   **In the larynx and associated structures:**
   A   the vocal cord is attached posteriorly via the vocal process to the arytenoid cartilage
   B   the cricoid cartilage articulates below with the thyroid cartilage and above with the arytenoids
   C   the cricothyroid ligament is an anterior thickening of the cricovocal membrane
   D   the hyoid bone is at the level of the third cervical vertebra
   E   the isthmus of the thyroid gland is just below the inferior border of the thyroid cartilage.

VIII.13   **The basilic vein:**
   A   is the continuation of the superficial palmar venous arch
   B   ascends initially on the posterior ulnar aspect of the forearm
   C   is related to the medial cutaneous nerve of forearm
   D   lies medial to biceps in the upper arm
   E   is a better route for a central venous catheter than the cephalic vein because it does not perforate the deep fascia.

VIII.14   **The trigeminal nerve:**
   A   is the largest cranial nerve
   B   provides sensation to most of the scalp
   C   provides somatic sensation to the eyeball
   D   provides sensation to the anterior two-thirds of the buccal mucosa
   E   supplies the muscles of mastication.

VIII.15   **An ankle block requires the application of local anaesthetic:**
   A   between the Achilles tendon and the medial malleolus
   B   between the Achilles tendon and the lateral malleolus
   C   anteriorly midway between the malleoli
   D   subcutaneously from the front of the tibia to the lateral malleolus
   E   to block the saphenous nerve.

VIII.16 **Serum electrolyte measurements of 125 mmol/l sodium and 6.2 mmol/l potassium are consistent with a diagnosis of:**
- A   acute renal failure
- B   hypopituitarism
- C   Addison's disease
- D   primary hyperaldosteronism
- E   Cushing's disease.

VIII.17 **Causes of right bundle branch block include:**
- A   pulmonary embolism
- B   myxoedema
- C   myocardial ischaemia
- D   myotonia congenita
- E   atrial septal defect.

VIII.18 **After an acute myocardial infarction, a patient is in sinus rhythm at 80 beats per minute and has a blood pressure of 110/70. Appropriate treatment for asymptomatic multifocal ventricular extrasystoles occurring at 10 per minute is:**
- A   atropine 600 µg intravenously
- B   propranolol 1 mg intravenously
- C   controlled 28% oxygen therapy
- D   lignocaine 100 mg intravenously
- E   flecainide 100 mg intravenously.

VIII.19 **A 68-year-old man, a known hypertensive taking metoprolol, is admitted to casualty with central chest pain. He is pale and sweaty and has a blood pressure of 70/50. The following are true :**
- A   a thrombolytic agent should be given as soon as possible in casualty
- B   analgesia should be withheld until there is a firm diagnosis
- C   verapamil is reasonable treatment for atrial fibrillation
- D   a high central venous pressure is diagnostic of poor left ventricular function
- E   he should be given a high concentration of oxygen by mask.

VIII.20 **Likely symptoms of diabetic ketoacidosis include:**
- A   hyperventilation
- B   extracellular dehydration
- C   extracellular sodium loss
- D   a hyperdynamic circulation
- E   coma.

VIII.21   **Acute gastrointestinal haemorrhage:**

   A   is mostly due to duodenal ulcer
   B   has a higher mortality when from gastric ulcers than from duodenal ulcers
   C   is a contraindication to any sedation
   D   increases serum creatinine
   E   is an indication for surgery when more than 4 units of blood have been given.

VIII.22   **In a patient with sickle cell disease, a crisis can be precipitated by:**

   A   suxamethonium
   B   hyperthermia
   C   acidosis
   D   enflurane
   E   hypoxia.

VIII.23   **The following can cause a spastic paraparesis:**

   A   multiple sclerosis
   B   subacute combined degeneration of the cord
   C   anterior spinal artery thrombosis
   D   diabetic neuropathy
   E   syringomyelia.

VIII.24   **Techniques that are suitable for use in patients with acute renal failure include:**

   A   brachial plexus block
   B   a propofol infusion
   C   spinal anaesthesia
   D   neuromuscular blockade with an infusion of atracurium
   E   intermittent positive pressure ventilation with isoflurane.

VIII.25   **Alveolar hypoventilation occurs if there is:**

   A   increased intracranial pressure
   B   emphysema
   C   pleural effusion
   D   asthma
   E   metabolic alkalosis.

VIII.26   The following are true of asthma:
A   the prognosis is not affected by age of onset
B   cromoglycate is of benefit in the acute attack
C   steroid treatment should be reserved for patients with severe asthma
D   mechanical ventilation is safe in the severe asthmatic and should be used to give the patient a good night's rest
E   the patient should be taught to match salbutamol usage to severity of symptoms.

VIII.27   Carcinoma of the large bowel:
A   is more common in Europeans than in Africans
B   will not have metastasised if it has not breached the serosal surface
C   is more common in the sigmoid colon than the transverse colon
D   can present with anaemia
E   is less likely to cause obstruction if in the ascending colon.

VIII.28   Appropriate conservative measures in the treatment of hiatus hernia include:
A   steroid therapy
B   anticholinergic therapy
C   weight loss
D   histamine (H_2) receptor antagonist therapy
E   omeprazole therapy.

VIII.29   Surgical hypophysectomy:
A   is usually by an extracranial approach
B   necessitates preoperative steroid therapy
C   can produce postoperative diabetes insipidus
D   requires both mineralocorticoid and glucocorticoid replacement postoperatively
E   is a contraindication to induced hypotension.

VIII.30   After elective hysterectomy, a 45-year-old patient is admitted to the intensive care unit cyanosed and with severe right-sided chest pain, sinus tachycardia and hypotension. Likely diagnoses include:
A   myocardial infarction
B   septicaemia
C   pulmonary embolism
D   bronchopneumonia
E   spontaneous pneumothorax.

Paper VIII Answers

VIII.1 FTTFF

A   There is no reason to change his current antihypertensive therapy if it is effective.

D   Intraoperative medication is not necessary unless there is hypertension or evidence of inadequate beta-adrenergic blockade.

E   There is no reason to restrict fluids unless there is cardiac failure – in which case beta-blockers are a poor choice of drug.

VIII.2 FFTTT

A   Stridor is a common presenting symptom.

B   The safest techniques are awake fibreoptic intubation, or tracheostomy under local anaesthesia.

C   An antisialogue is not essential, but many patients with advanced laryngeal cancer find swallowing difficult and tend to drool.

D   These are vagal effects caused by pressure on the carotid bifurcation.

E   Parathyroid damage can occur during surgery.

VIII.3 TTFTF

C   Susceptible individuals must have their temperature monitored, but the rise in temperature may be delayed and the diagnosis can be made from many of the other signs (rigidity, increased carbon dioxide output, and so on).

D   The urine is coloured by myoglobin.

E   Always read doses carefully. The usual dose of dantrolene is 1–10 mg/kg; 4 mg/kg is the typical dose to control a reaction.

VIII.4 FFFFT

A   In severe tracheal stenosis the low density of helium/oxygen mixtures may ease ventilation of the patient, but nitrous oxide is not contraindicated.

B,D Although in both cases, nitrous oxide will diffuse into the cavities, it would not increase pressure enough to cause a problem. How many times have you yourself used nitrous oxide for large bowel surgery?

C   The leak may make ventilation difficult, but does not affect the leak.

E   The cyst might enlarge and rupture.

VIII.5   **FTTFF**

A,D,   Although all these complications have been reported
E   and, indeed, almost anything can happen, the key word in the question is 'likely', and likely complications of the infraclavicular approach are **B,C**.

VIII.6   **FTFFT**

A   Vasospasm is common postoperatively and may cause neurological deficits.
B   Nimodipine has been licensed for this use.
D   It is often better for assessment to have the patient awake.

VIII.7   **TFFTF**

B   Glycopyrronium is an anticholinergic with no useful effect on acidity.
C   Metoclopramide speeds gastric emptying but cannot neutralise gastric acid.
D   Ranitidine raises gastric pH and volume if given well before the operation. Antacid should be given as well.
E   Omeprazole blocks the proton pump, and at the time of writing has just been licensed for obstetric use.

VIII.8   **FTTTF**

A   This sign is associated with retroperitoneal haemorrhage. It occurs in pancreatitis.
C   Intra-abdominal bleeding can cause bradycardia rather than the expected tachycardia of hypovolaemia.
E   Sweating is not a feature of a ruptured ectopic pregnancy.

VIII.9   **TFTFF**

B   Skin blood flow is decreased by the vasoconstriction of sympathetic activity.
C   Skin blood flow increases in the segments blocked by the epidural. The upper limbs may vasoconstrict in compensation.
D   Thiopentone causes peripheral vasodilation.
E   Skin blood flow decreases in most low output states.

VIII.10   **TTFFF**

C,E   Both phenylbutazone and phenytoin can precipitate an acute attack.
D   Barbiturates are the classical drug cause of an acute attack of porphyria.

VIII.11   TFFTF

  B   Nitrogen washout is a method (now old-fashioned) for measuring the anatomical dead space.

  C   The patient may depend on hypoxic drive, but this is not a useful clinical test.

  E   The main problem is obstruction, not diffusion. Anaesthetic gases are very soluble and their uptake is not clinically influenced by alterations in the transfer factor.

VIII.12   TTTTF

  The anatomy of the larynx is difficult to visualise: try to find a three-dimensional model to study.

  C,E   This is the site for emergency puncture. The isthmus lies inferior to the cricoid cartilage, overlying the second to fourth tracheal rings.

VIII.13   FTTTF

  A   The basilic vein drains the ulnar dorsal venous network.

  B   It becomes anterior before it reaches the elbow.

  E   It is a better route than the cephalic vein, because catheters stick where the cephalic vein perforates the clavi-pectoral fascia. But the basilic vein does perforate the deep fascia – midway up the upper arm.

VIII.14   TFTFT

  B   The trigeminal supplies the scalp to the vertex. Posterior to the vertex is supplied by the occipital nerves via the cervical plexus.

  D   The trigeminal supplies the anterior two-thirds of the *tongue*, but the whole of the mouth, gums and palate.

VIII.15   TTTTT

  Five parts of an MCQ = five nerves to be blocked for a successful ankle block: **A** the posterior tibial nerve, **B** the sural nerve, **C** the anterior tibial nerve, **D** the musculocutaneous nerve, and **E** the saphenous nerve (blocked just superior to the medial malleolus).

VIII.16   TTTFF

D   Hyperaldosteronism will promote sodium retention and potassium loss.

E   Sodium is retained in Cushing's disease.

VIII.17   TFTFT

B,D   Right bundle branch block is not associated with myxoedema or myotonia congenita.

VIII.18   FFFTF

A   Atropine is suitable only for ventricular ectopics occurring as escape beats.

B   Propranolol may make ectopics worse.

C   There is no reason to withhold higher concentrations of oxygen if oxygen is indicated.

E   A multicentre trial showed that flecainide doubles the mortality in these patients.

VIII.19   FFFFT

A   Early thrombolysis is desirable after an infarct but from the information we are given he might have a dissected thoracic aneurysm or had a pulmonary embolism. At the least, an electrocardiogram is required.

B   Analgesia is both humane and therapeutic; morphine is good treatment for heart failure.

C   Verapamil is reasonable treatment – but can precipitate asystole with beta-blockers.

D   A high venous pressure may indicate a problem on the right side of the heart.

E   Yes, though all too often he will be given a Ventimask!

VIII.20   TTTFT

D   The circulation tends to be hypodynamic.

VIII.21   FTFFF

Note that the site of bleeding is not defined, it just says 'gastrointestinal', and therefore covers both haematemesis and melaena.

A   This is even less 'true' now, because of the H_2 antagonists.

D   Urea, but not the creatinine, is increased by absorption of blood.

E   Surgery is required less frequently now that the range of endoscopic treatments is greater.

VIII.22   FFTFT

A   Suxamethonium can cause many problems but does not precipitate sickle cell crisis unless indirectly via hypoxia caused by failed intubation.

B   Hypothermia is a risk factor.

D   Volatile anaesthetics are not risk factors unless severe cardiorespiratory depression produces either profound hypotension or acidosis.

VIII.23   TTFFT

A   Multiple sclerosis is a cause, especially in middle-aged women.

C   Spinal artery thrombosis causes acute flaccid paralysis.

E   Upper limb signs are much more obvious in syringomyelia.

VIII.24   TTTTT

B   Propofol is converted to inactive metabolites in the liver.

D   There have been concerns about accumulation of the metabolite laudanosine in patients with renal failure given infusions of atracurium, but it is not a problem clinically.

VIII.25   TTTTT

A   Raised intracranial pressure, if raised enough, causes depression of the medullary respiratory centre.

D   Asthma causes hyperventilation initially but in severe cases eventually there will be alveolar hypoventilation, and $PaCO_2$ will increase.

E   Hypoventilation is compensation for the alkalosis.

VIII.26 FFFFF

    A   Most children grow out of their asthma, and suffer fewer symptoms than adults.

    B   Cromoglycate is sometimes useful for prophylaxis of mild asthma and exercise-induced asthma. It does not help an acute attack.

    C   The 1993 British Thoracic Society guidelines recommend use of inhaled steroids for patients with moderately severe asthma.

    D   The incidence of barotrauma is high in the asthmatic.

    E   Excessive use by patients of adrenergic bronchodilators during acute attacks can cause overdosage, as well as delaying treatment with steroids. Patients must be taught not to use their inhalers too often, and it is steroid therapy that should be increased in exacerbations.

VIII.27 TFTTT

    B   Less likely to have metastasised, perhaps, but cancer does not follow rules.

    D   Anaemia is the presenting symptom especially when the tumour is in the caecum or ascending colon.

    E   The faeces are less solid in the ascending colon.

VIII.28 FFTTT

    B   Anticholinergics may be used in achalasia, but not usually in hiatus hernia.

VIII.29 TTTTF

    E   Elective intraoperative hypotension can be used.

VIII.30 FFTTT

Note that there is no mention of how long it is since the operation.

    A   Infarction is not likely: premenopausal, and right-sided pain.

    B   Generalised septicaemia should not cause chest pain.

    C,D At 10 days, pulmonary embolism is the most likely; bronchopneumonia must also be considered but is more likely earlier.

    E   This is the most likely if shortly after operation.

Paper IX   Questions

IX.1   **A patient suddenly complains of pain in the arm during induction of anaesthesia with 2.5% thiopentone:**
A   the patient should be reassured
B   20 mg lignocaine should be added to the injection
C   the patient may have suffered a myocardial infarct
D   there is likely to be evidence of local histamine release
E   anaphylaxis is likely.

IX.2   **A maturity onset diabetic presents for repair of an inguinal hernia. He is taking an oral hypoglycaemic. Suitable preparation for anaesthesia and surgery includes:**
A   setting up an intravenous infusion of 5% dextrose if the blood sugar is less than 3 mmol/l
B   omitting the normal dose of oral hypoglycaemic on the morning of operation
C   giving the normal dose of oral hypoglycaemic on the morning of operation and a single injection of 25 g dextrose immediately before anaesthesia
D   deleting the morning dose of oral hypoglycaemic and giving 12 units of Actrapid insulin intravenously before anaesthesia
E   setting up an infusion of 10% glucose 500 ml + 15 mmol KCl + 15 units Actrapid insulin at 100 ml/h when the patient arrives in the anaesthetic room.

IX.3   Intraocular pressure is increased by:
A   hyperventilation
B   hypoxia
C   atropine premedication
D   suxamethonium
E   acetazolamide.

IX.4   Allowing for blood loss into sucker bottles, blood loss during operation is accurately assessed:
A   by careful monitoring of the central venous pressure
B   by weighing swabs
C   by washing swabs and towels in water and measuring the resulting haemoglobin concentration
D   from the haematocrit
E   from the total buffer base.

IX.5   Features of acute fat embolism include:
A   unilateral tremor of the hand
B   pyrexia
C   carbon dioxide retention
D   petechial haemorrhages
E   retinal oedema.

IX.6   High epidural anaesthesia to T1 impairs cardiac performance by:
A   slowing the heart
B   reducing venous return
C   reducing sensitivity to endogenous adrenaline
D   lowering serum cortisol response to stress
E   reducing the left ventricular ejection fraction.

IX.7   **Agents suitable for elective hypotension during surgery for an intracranial aneurysm include:**
A   sodium nitroprusside
B   phenoxybenzamine
C   trimetaphan
D   isoflurane
E   isosorbide dinitrate.

IX.8   **Contraindications to the use of epidural anaesthesia for vaginal delivery include:**
A   placenta praevia
B   hypovolaemia
C   breech presentation
D   unengaged fetal head
E   pre-eclampsia.

IX.9   **Chronic deep pain:**
A   is unrelieved by spino-thalamic tractotomy
B   is characteristically made worse by transcutaneous nerve stimulation
C   can be relieved by midbrain stimulation
D   is made worse by cutting peripheral nerves
E   indicates underlying organic pathology of the central nervous system.

IX.10   **Adequate premedication with opioids:**
A   reduces the amount of induction agent required
B   increases plasma cortisol levels
C   suppresses beta-adrenergic activity
D   releases enkephalin antagonists in the midbrain
E   causes nausea and vomiting.

IX.11   **Appropriate preventative measures in a patient thought to have suffered an anaphylactic reaction during a previous anaesthetic include:**
A   antihistamine premedication
B   preoperative disodium cromoglycate
C   induction with etomidate
D   the avoidance of suxamethonium
E   complement stabilisation with indomethacin.

IX.12   Appropriate treatment for a supraventricular tachycardia occurring after pneumonectomy includes:

A   intravenous propranolol
B   carotid sinus massage
C   intramuscular digoxin
D   synchronised DC shock
E   intravenous adenosine.

IX.13   Block of the brachial plexus by the axillary route:

A   has no complications
B   provides complete analgesia of the forearm
C   is contraindicated in sickle-cell disease
D   will not allow manipulation of a dislocated shoulder
E   occasionally misses the musculocutaneous nerve.

IX.14   The following are true of the posterior primary rami in the thoracic and lumbar regions:

A   they all divide into medial and lateral branches
B   they form plexuses to supply the backs of the upper arms and backs of the thighs
C   the skin over the iliac crest is supplied by T12
D   the lateral branches of L1–3 supply skin
E   the lateral branches of L4–5 supply the skin up to but not including the skin surrounding the anal margin.

IX.15   The lumbar plexus:

A   forms within the body of psoas major
B   may receive a contribution from T12
C   is normally L1 to L5
D   supplies sensation to the whole of the anteromedial aspect of the thigh
E   is formed by the anterior primary rami.

IX.16   Situations likely to result in the development of acute hyperkalaemia include:

A   malignant hyperpyrexia
B   adrenocortical insufficiency
C   triamterene therapy
D   crush injuries
E   anabolic steroid therapy.

IX.17 **Likely causes of left bundle branch block include:**
A ischaemic heart disease
B cardiomyopathy
C diabetes mellitus
D digitalis therapy
E mitral incompetence.

IX.18 **In the jugular venous pulse:**
A the 'a' wave corresponds to atrial systole
B the 'y' descent follows opening of the AV valves
C giant 'a' waves occur in pulmonary hypertension
D a large 'v' wave occurs in tricuspid incompetence
E cannon waves occur in tricuspid stenosis.

IX.19 **Functional consequences of moderately severe mitral stenosis include:**
A decreased pulmonary compliance
B an increase in left atrial pressure
C hypercapnia at rest
D an increase in the left ventricular end-diastolic pressure
E a decrease in glomerular filtration rate.

IX.20 **The emergency treatment of myxoedema coma includes:**
A intravenous hydrocortisone
B intravenous thyroxine
C intravenous saline
D aqueous oral iodine (Lugol's solution)
E rapid warming.

IX.21 **Causes of portal hypertension include:**
A neonatal umbilical sepsis
B haemochromatosis
C Budd–Chiari syndrome
D anaemia
E alpha$_1$-antitrypsin deficiency.

IX.22 **Likely causes of a bleeding disorder that first becomes apparent during surgery include:**
A acute fibrinogenaemia
B prothrombin deficiency
C plasminogen activation
D von Willebrand's disease
E sickle cell disease.

IX.23 Petit mal epilepsy:
A   commonly causes syncope
B   is most common after puberty
C   is precipitated by overbreathing
D   usually leads to mental retardation
E   has a characteristic EEG pattern.

IX.24 Prednisolone:
A   is used in the treatment of Addison's disease
B   causes gastric ulceration
C   causes hyperkalaemia
D   produces osteoporosis
E   causes hyponatraemia.

IX.25 Toxic effects of oxygen therapy include:
A   corneal ulceration
B   reduced pulmonary diffusing capacity
C   retrolental fibroplasia
D   convulsions
E   pulmonary vasoconstriction.

IX.26 A 57-year-old alcoholic is admitted to hospital with intermittent pyrexia, dyspnoea and copious sputum from which staphylococcus is cultured. A chest radiograph shows an opacity in the right middle zone with a fluid level. Appropriate treatment includes:
A   diagnostic transpleural aspiration
B   thoracotomy and lobectomy
C   postural drainage
D   drainage via an underwater seal
E   intravenous antibiotics.

IX.27 The following occur in acute pancreatitis:
A   retroperitoneal haemorrhage
B   tetany
C   pancreatic abscess
D   pseudocyst formation
E   hyperglycaemia.

IX.28 Primary malignant tumours which commonly metastasise to bone include:
A   uterine carcinoma
B   rhabdomyosarcoma
C   gastric carcinoma
D   testicular teratoma
E   prostatic carcinoma.

IX.29 At an out-patient appointment following gastrectomy for a benign gastric tumour, a 49-year-old man complains of dizziness that comes on an hour or two after meals. The following are true:

A   the dizziness is likely to be relieved by food
B   the dizziness is likely to be accompanied by nausea
C   the patient should be investigated for insulinoma
D   an anastomotic ulcer is likely
E   he may be helped by taking a short-acting hypoglycaemic drug before meals.

IX.30 The following are true of tumours of the testicle:

A   trauma is a predisposing factor
B   the most common presentation is an enlarged testicle
C   most seminomas are radiosensitive
D   gynaecomastia is a rare feature
E   they may be part of the pluriglandular syndrome.

Paper IX Answers

IX.1 TFFTF

A The danger of intra-arterial injection of thiopentone is well known. It is far less likely now that we rarely induce anaesthesia via a simple needle but usually site an intravenous cannula. Whatever is happening – even if anaphylaxis is developing to a drug – the patient should always be reassured.

B Lignocaine reduces the pain of injecting etomidate, methohexitone and propofol, but forms a precipitate with thiopentone.

C It is easy to invent convoluted scenarios when answering MCQs. A typical scenario here would be: intravenous thiopentone causes hypotension – hypotension reduces coronary filling – a patient may have a myocardial infarction. But this is scarcely a likely possibility – added to which the hypotensive effect of thiopentone occurs after unconsciousness.

E Anaphylaxis occurs in about one in 20 000–25 000 administrations of thiopentone. Pain is not a premonitory symptom.

IX.2 FTFFT

The perioperative control of diabetes is an obvious and important question in anaesthesia examinations (see Q V.2).

A The patient is at risk of hypoglycaemia. A higher concentration of glucose is needed.

C Oral hypoglycaemics must be withdrawn the day before operation; a single dose of intravenous glucose will not cover for the prolonged effect of the oral drug.

D Just giving a single dose of insulin without glucose, especially without measurement of the blood glucose, is likely to cause hypoglycaemia.

E An insulin/glucose/potassium regimen may not be necessary, but would be a suitable method of treatment if the patient were poorly controlled on oral hypoglycaemics.

IX.3   FTFTF

A   *Hyper*ventilation (hypocapnia) decreases intraocular pressure.

B   Hypoxia can cause hypertension, and blood pressure is an important determinant of intraocular pressure.

C   Atropine in the normal premedicant dose does not affect intraocular pressure in the normal eye.

E   Acetazolamide is a carbonic anhydrase inhibitor. It reduces intraocular pressure by reducing the formation of aqueous humour.

IX.4   FFTFF

Accurate assessment of intraoperative blood loss is difficult.

A   The central venous pressure is notoriously unhelpful in young, fit adults. Once a patient is already hypovolaemic the central venous pressure is a useful guide to fluid *replacement* – but that is not the same as knowing how much blood has been *lost*.

B,C   Weighing swabs is a *guide* to blood loss, but is not accurate; swabs may become saturated with irrigation fluids. Washing swabs in a known volume of water is the most accurate technique we have. It is often used in research, and is sometimes used in neonatal practice, but it is cumbersome.

D   The patient's intraoperative haemoglobin concentration and haematocrit are rough guides only.

E   Haemoglobin is part of the total buffer base, but total buffer base is of no use.

IX.5   FTTTF

A   The cerebral symptoms of acute fat embolism are mainly those of cerebral hypoxia. There may be fitting.

C   Carbon dioxide is retained because of impaired pulmonary gas exchange.

E   Fat may be seen in the retinal vessels. Retinal oedema is not a characteristic.

IX.6   TTFFF

C   High epidural anaesthesia denervates the adrenal glands and therefore reduces adrenaline output, but does not have any effect on the myocardial sensitivity to catecholamines.

E   Left ventricular ejection fraction is not affected by epidural anaesthesia in the normal myocardium.

IX.7   TFTTF

B   Phenoxybenzamine is a long-acting alpha-adrenergic blocker, unsuitable for readily controllable surgical hypotension.

C   Trimetaphan used to be a popular hypotensive drug. Some still use it, though the dilated pupils can be worrying.

D   Isoflurane is often used in combination with another agent.

E   The hypotension produced by isosorbide is usually insufficient for neurosurgery.

IX.8   FTFFF

A   The development of high quality scans has made it easier to assess placenta praevia. If the obstetrician attempts vaginal delivery an epidural is suitable, though a caesarean section is more likely.

C   Regional anaesthesia is often used to allow assisted delivery of a breech presentation. There are curious regional variations. In the UK, breech presentation is an indication for an epidural. In some parts of Europe it is a relative contraindication.

D   The fetal head may engage only late in labour. Painful contractions may occur earlier in labour.

E   Epidurals are indicated (provided clotting is normal).

IX.9   TFTTF

A   The spinothalamic tracts carry only cutaneous pain.

B   TENS may help to relieve the pain.

E   Any pain can have many causes, including psychological ones.

IX.10   TFFFT

Opioid premedication is used less than it used to be. Its benefits should not be forgotten.

B   Opioids certainly do not increase cortisol levels. They may lessen the stress-induced increases.

C   There is no effect on beta-adrenergic activity.

D   There is no evidence that enkephalin antagonists are released.

IX.11   TTTTF

B   Antihistamine premedication stabilises mast cells and blocks effects of released histamine.

C   Etomidate is the least likely of the induction agents to cause anaphylactic-type reactions.

E   There is no evidence that indomethacin stabilises complement or should be used as prophylaxis.

IX.12   TTFTT

There is nothing special about treating a supraventricular tachycardia just because it has occurred after pneumonectomy – except that you should always think of some specific trigger. Is a chest drain or a central venous catheter touching the heart?

A   Propranolol is not now a first line of treatment. Remember that patients needing pneumonectomy may have some heart failure, be taking calcium channel antagonists or have reversible airways disease – all of which demand caution when giving beta-blocking drugs.

C   Digoxin is long-term treatment for atrial fibrillation. Otherwise it is not appropriate here.

E   Adenosine is probably the safest initial drug, as it allows more accurate diagnosis, is evanescent, and causes less cardiac depression than drugs such as verapamil.

IX.13   FTFTT

A   The axillary approach is certainly less hazardous than the more proximal approaches, but nerve damage and intravascular injection of anaesthetic can occur.

B,E   Note that these are not mutually exclusive.

C   A tourniquet is contraindicated, but not the block itself.

IX.14   TFTTF

A   Beware thinking that nothing is 'always' or 'never' in medicine. The posterior rami all divide into medial and lateral branches.

B   Plexuses are formed by the *anterior* primary rami.

E   L4–5 do not supply skin.

IX.15   TTFTT

C   The lumbar plexus is normally L1 to L4.

D   T12 supplies the skin over the lateral buttock (subcostal nerve) and iliac crest (posterior primary ramus) but that is not 'anteromedial'.

IX.16   TTTTF

A   Potassium is released as muscle cells break down.

B   Adrenocortical insufficiency causes hyponatraemia and hyperkalaemia.

C   Triamterene is a potassium-conserving diuretic that can cause hyperkalaemia if used inadvisedly.

E   Anabolic steroids do not cause hyperkalaemia.

IX.17   TTFTF

A,C   Left bundle branch block is most commonly caused by ischaemic heart disease, which is more likely in diabetics, but diabetes is not associated with bundle branch block.

E   Aortic but not mitral valve disease is a cause of left bundle branch block.

IX.18   TTTTF

E   Cannon waves occur in tricuspid incompetence, not stenosis.

IX.19   TTFFT

It would be interesting to ask a number of cardiologists what was meant by 'moderately severe' mitral stenosis, but questions with similar wording do crop up in exams, so you will have to make up your mind.

C   Hypercapnia implies hypoventilation or reduced drive to ventilation.

D   The left ventricle is beyond the stenosed valve and so its end-diastolic pressure will not be affected.

E   We are assuming that moderately severe disease means that there is some heart failure, so glomerular filtration will be reduced.

IX.20   TFTFF

B   Intravenous T3 (triiodothyronine) is given in myxoedema coma, not thyroxine.

C   Patients must be rehydrated carefully, to avoid heart failure.

D   Lugol's iodine is used to treat thyrotoxicosis.

E   Patients must be rewarmed slowly. Rapid rewarming may cause arrhythmias, hypovolaemia and hypoglycaemia.

IX.21   TTTFT

B   Severe liver disease is a late and potentially preventable manifestation of primary haemochromatosis.

C   Budd–Chiari syndrome produces a hyperdynamic systemic circulation, but not portal hypertension.

E   Alpha$_1$-antitrypsin deficiency is a rare cause of cirrhosis. Patients also have emphysema.

IX.22   TTTTF

E   Sickle cell disease causes problems because of the formation of peripheral microemboli but it is not a bleeding disorder.

IX.23   FFFFT

A   In petit mal epilepsy patients go blank for a few moments ('little absences') but do not usually fall down.

B   It is commoner before puberty and tends to regress in later life.

C   Overbreathing causes hypocapnia, which is a cause of cerebral irritability that can precipitate epileptiform convulsions in susceptible patients. Petit mal has a different mechanism.

D   Frequent petit mal attacks may cause learning difficulties despite normal intelligence.

IX.24   TTFTF

C,E   Corticosteroid therapy causes hypokalaemia and sodium retention.

IX.25   FTTTT

A   Corneal ulceration is a complication only of direct application of oxygen to the eyes.

D   Convulsions occur at pressures of oxygen above 2 atmospheres absolute. This branch is 'true' because the question asks generally for all 'included' toxic effects and does not specify normal atmospheric pressure.

IX.26   TFTFT

A   Ultrasound-guided percutaneous aspiration would allow determination of bacterial antibiotic sensitivity.

B   Thoracotomy is not needed unless conservative treatment fails.

D   Drainage is needed only for an associated bronchopleural fistula.

IX.27   TTTTT

IX.28   FTTFT

Note inclusion of the word 'commonly'.

A   Uterine carcinoma spreads locally and transperitoneally.

D   Testicular teratoma spreads intra-abdominally.

IX.29   TTFFF

The patient is likely to be suffering from late-dumping syndrome, which is caused by hypoglycaemia.

C   Insulinoma is rare and often missed – but there is no reason to suspect one here.

D   Dizziness after meals is not a symptom of anastomotic ulcer.

E   Hypoglycaemic drugs may help in *early* dumping.

IX.30   FTTTF

A   Trauma may draw the patient's attention to the swelling, and undescended testes (which are more liable to trauma) are more likely to become malignant. Trauma is not in itself a factor.

Paper X Questions

X.1 **Likely causes of hypotension developing during chair dental surgery are:**
    A emotional factors
    B hypoxia secondary to obstruction from the dental pack
    C carotid sinus pressure
    D vagal blockade
    E blood loss.

X.2 **During anaesthesia for middle ear surgery:**
    A moderate elective hypotension is essential
    B beta-adrenergic blocking agents should not be used
    C air embolism is likely to occur
    D nitrous oxide administration should be discontinued at least 30 minutes before application of the graft
    E positive end-expiratory pressure (PEEP) helps reduce blood loss when there is moderate hypotension.

X.3 **Suitable treatment for intense peripheral vasoconstriction includes:**
    A intravenous phentolamine
    B sodium nitroprusside
    C propranolol
    D dobutamine
    E high spinal analgesia.

X.4   Factors predisposing to passive regurgitation include:
A   suxamethonium fasciculations
B   obesity
C   head injury
D   hiccoughs
E   preoperative metoclopramide.

X.5   During parenteral nutrition:
A   sorbitol therapy may cause a lactic acidosis
B   the normal daily potassium requirement is
     15–30 mmol/24 h
C   ethanol yields 7 calories per gram
D   utilisation of amino-acid solutions requires administration of
     glucose
E   more than 10% of infused insulin is adsorbed on to the
     plastic of the intravenous giving set.

**X.6   End-tidal carbon dioxide concentrations during neurosurgical
anaesthesia:**
A   vary with the depth of anaesthesia
B   are decreased by air embolism
C   should be kept at less than 3.0 kPa
D   increase at craniotomy
E   are decreased when there are large cerebral arteriovenous
     malformations.

X.7   **Suitable techniques for relieving pain in labour include:**
A   transcutaneous electrical nerve stimulation (TENS)
B   isoflurane via a draw-over vaporiser
C   epidural bupivacaine
D   aromatherapy
E   70% nitrous oxide in oxygen.

X.8   **In a neonate suspected of having a tracheo-oesophageal fistula:**
A   cyanosis is likely from birth
B   the cardinal sign is saliva pouring continuously from the mouth
C   a plain radiograph shows no air in the bowel
D   barium contrast media are absolutely contraindicated
E   it is probable that both stomach and upper oesophagus are joined to the trachea.

X.9   **Midazolam:**
A   is contraindicated in hepatic disease
B   is the best intravenous drug for providing anaesthesia for cardioversion
C   is a suitable agent for the sedation of patients with head injuries
D   is suitable for use in asthmatics
E   produces epileptiform changes on the EEG in susceptible individuals.

X.10   **Drugs known to increase tone in the sphincter of Oddi include:**
A   atropine
B   droperidol
C   morphine
D   glycopyrronium
E   fentanyl.

X.11   **A 30-year-old woman is admitted conscious after a suspected serious overdose of aspirin. Results of an arterial blood sample taken before treatment, with her breathing air, compatible with this diagnosis are:**

A   pH of 6.9
B $PaCO_2$ of 3.3 kPa (25 mmHg)
C PaO_2 of 10.1 kPa (76 mmHg)
D   standard bicarbonate of 11 mmol/l
E   base excess of −4 mmol/l.

X.12   **The following structures are related to the trachea at the level of the fourth thoracic vertebra:**

A   the aortic arch on the left
B   the mediastinal pleura on the right
C   the thoracic duct posteriorly on the left
D   the right recurrent laryngeal nerve
E   the right phrenic nerve.

X.13   **The following are true of the stellate ganglion:**

A   it is formed by the inferior cervical ganglion and the first thoracic ganglion
B   it supplies sympathetic fibres to the head, neck and upper arm
C   it can be blocked with 10 ml of 1% lignocaine at the level of the sixth or seventh cervical vertebrae
D   block causes an ipsilateral Horner's syndrome
E   during the block the patient should breathe slowly and deeply.

X.14   **The maxillary division of the trigeminal nerve:**

A   passes through the foramen rotundum
B   passes through the pterygopalatine fossa
C   receives the greater superficial petrosal nerve at the sphenopalatine ganglion
D   can be blocked by an approach on to the lateral pterygoid plate
E   has no motor components.

X.15   **In the neck:**

A   the internal jugular vein lies lateral to the common carotid artery in most patients
B   the oesophagus is separated from the vertebrae by the prevertebral fascia
C   the vagus nerves lie between the trachea and oesophagus
D   the sympathetic chain is immediately posterior to the common carotid sheath
E   the subclavian and internal jugular veins form the innominate (brachiocephalic) vein.

X.16   The following concentrations, in plasma from venous blood, are compatible with which of the conditions? Na$^+$ 127 mmol/l, K$^+$ 6.0 mmol/l, Cl$^-$ 85 mmol/l, HCO$_3^-$ 18 mmol/l, urea 18 mmol/l:
A   adrenocortical insufficiency
B   hepatic failure
C   renal failure
D   carcinoma of the lung with inappropriate ADH secretion
E   high small bowel obstruction with vomiting.

X.17   In a patient with acute myocardial infarction, the following sites of injury result in the following electrocardiographic changes:
A   in anteroseptal infarction, ST elevation and T wave inversion in lead I
B   in inferior infarction, ST elevation and T wave inversion in leads II, III and aVF
C   in subendocardial infarction, ST depression in the chest leads overlying the affected muscle
D   in anterolateral infarction, ST elevation in leads II, III, and aVL
E   in posterior infarction, ST elevation in lead I and aVR.

X.18   A patient with infective endocarditis suddenly becomes dyspnoeic, with a blood pressure of 130/50. The venous pressure is increased and systolic and diastolic murmurs become more pronounced. Likely diagnoses include:
A   pulmonary embolism
B   inferior myocardial infarction
C   prolapsed mitral valve cusp
D   aortic valve rupture
E   dissecting aortic aneurysm.

X.19   Clinical features suggestive of a VIPoma include:
A   hyperkalaemia
B   steatorrhoea
C   profuse watery diarrhoea
D   hypercalcaemia
E   acidosis.

X.20   Symptoms of hyperthyroidism likely to occur in a 25-year-old woman include:
A   reduced pulse pressure
B   lid lag
C   cold intolerance
D   menorrhagia
E   a thyroid bruit.

X.21   Weight loss with a normal appetite occurs in:

A   gastric carcinoma
B   Addison's disease
C   diabetes mellitus
D   thyrotoxicosis
E   tuberculosis.

X.22   Massive transfusion of stored ACD (acid-citrate-dextrose) blood results in:

A   a decrease in the plasma ionised calcium
B   a metabolic, non-respiratory, acidosis
C   thrombocytopenia
D   hyponatraemia
E   hypokalaemia.

X.23   The effects of infused noradrenaline are potentiated in:

A   Horner's syndrome
B   peripheral neuropathy
C   sepsis syndrome
D   treatment with guanethidine
E   patients undergoing lumbar extradural anaesthesia.

X.24   In the first 3 days after major abdominal surgery, there is reduced urinary excretion of:

A   potassium
B   sodium
C   nitrogen
D   water
E   chloride.

X.25   In an emphysematous patient of the 'pink puffer' type:

A   onset of dyspnoea occurs late in life
B   alveolar gas transfer is reduced
C   polycythaemia is common
D   a chest X-ray shows normal vascular markings
E   cor pulmonale is a frequent occurrence.

X.26   **Signs of acute hypoxia include:**
    A   muscular rigidity
    B   miosis
    C   irregular breathing
    D   slow, bounding pulse
    E   extraocular muscle spasm.

X.27   **The following are true of occlusive vascular disease of the large blood vessels of the legs:**
    A   it occurs predominantly in cigarette smokers
    B   oral vasodilators are effective temporary treatment for intermittent claudication
    C   50% of patients will eventually die of direct complications such as gangrene
    D   associated coronary vessel disease is uncommon
    E   distal flow after surgery can be assessed using a pulse oximeter.

X.28   **Indications for laparotomy following suspected abdominal injury include:**
    A   tachycardia in the absence of hypotension
    B   left shoulder tip pain
    C   abdominal distension in the absence of obvious signs of haemorrhage
    D   free gas under the right diaphragm
    E   bruising of the loin and dullness to percussion of the flanks.

X.29   **Indications for operative intervention in the first hour after a head injury include:**
    A   diminishing level of consciousness
    B   unilateral pupillary dilation
    C   respiratory arrest
    D   CSF rhinorrhoea
    E   generalised convulsions.

X.30   **In a patient suspected of suffering from porphyria and about to undergo anaesthesia and surgery for acute appendicitis:**
    A   propofol is a safe intravenous induction agent
    B   isoflurane is contraindicated
    C   serum sodium and potassium concentrations are low
    D   blood urea may be increased
    E   non-depolarising neuromuscular blocking drugs should not be used.

Paper X Answers

X.1 **TTTFF**

A Induction of anaesthesia in an anxious patient reduces the previously high sympathetic drive.

B We hope that your superb technique and the use of a pulse oximeter will prevent hypoxia. Hypoxia can cause bradycardia and hypotension, especially in children, though classically hypertension is supposed to occur first.

C,D Pressure during jaw support can cause inadvertent pressure on the carotid sinus. This is an example of vagal *stimulation*, and causes bradycardia.

E Blood loss sufficient to cause hypotension is unlikely during chair dental surgery.

X.2 **FFFFF**

A Induced hypotension may reduce bleeding and make surgery easier and quicker, but the advantages of the technique must be balanced against the risk to the patient.

B Beta-blockers are often used as part of the hypotensive technique.

C An air embolus is extremely unlikely unless the mastoids are involved.

D Nitrous oxide should be discontinued if the graft is *overlaid*. It doesn't matter if the graft is *underlaid*, which is the more common technique nowadays.

E PEEP is inappropriate. If the patient has already been given hypotensive agents, PEEP may cause severe hypotension. Also, the increase in venous pressure may make grafting more difficult.

X.3 **TTFFF**

Remember that you must be aware of the circulating volume before giving potent vasodilators.

C Beta-blockers *cause* peripheral vasoconstriction.

D If dobutamine is given to hypovolaemic patients, the resulting peripheral vasodilation can reduce blood pressure, but dobutamine has little effect on intense vasoconstriction.

E High spinal analgesia causes peripheral vasodilation but is scarcely a suitable technique.

X.4   TTFTF

D   Hiccoughs, for instance associated with propofol anaesthesia, produce measurable regurgitation, although it is probably not clinically important.

E   Metoclopramide increases barrier pressure and therefore should reduce the risk of regurgitation.

X.5   TFTTT

B   You can assume this is a 'standard' adult. The normal daily potassium requirement is 40–60 mmol per day.

D   Utilisation of amino-acids needs glucose: the balance should be 200 kcal/g (48 kJ/g) nitrogen.

X.6   FTFFF

A   There is some evidence that, in general, less anaesthetic is needed at lower carbon dioxide concentrations. There is no suggestion that the depth of anaesthesia has any effect on carbon dioxide.

B   End-tidal carbon dioxide concentrations decrease because of increased dead space (lung that is ventilated but not perfused).

C   Vasoconstriction causes cerebral anaerobic metabolism at much below 4.0 kPa.

D   Opening the skull has no effect. The body's carbon dioxide is a balance between metabolism and alveolar ventilation: craniotomy should have no effect. Insufficient analgesia as the skull is opened *could* increase the metabolic rate (because of increased sympathetic drive), but whereas the haemodynamic effects of this are obvious, any possible effects on carbon dioxide are not.

E   There is no reason why arteriovenous malformations should affect end-tidal carbon dioxide.

X.7   TFTFF

A   TENS is effective for some women in early labour.
B   This technique could be used, although in practice it is
     not. The last volatile agent widely used for pain relief in
     labour was methoxyflurane in the 1970s. The OMV
     (Oxford Miniature Vaporizer) is the only calibrated
     draw-over isoflurane vaporiser.
C   Surely there are few who will not mark this 'true' – but it
     is salutary that there are few properly controlled trials
     comparing epidurals with other methods of pain relief in
     labour that have looked at all aspects of the treatments
     (pain relief, effect on labour and longer-term side effects).
D   Aromatherapy produces a nice ambience and a relaxed
     patient (in those who want it), but it is not effective at
     treating established painful contractions.
E   Entonox is 50% nitrous oxide. The higher concentration of
     70% causes loss of consciousness in most subjects. It is
     not suitable for use during labour.

X.8   FTFTF

A   Coughing and cyanosis occur on feeding, which is
     contraindicated once the diagnosis is made. Delayed
     diagnosis may cause cyanosis secondary to aspiration.
C   A stomach full of air is a sign of the condition.
E   This is the least common presentation of the
     malformation. Generally the upper oesophagus is a blind
     pouch and the stomach joins the lower trachea.

X.9   FFTTF

A   Dose should be reduced, but is not contraindicated.
B   Benzodiazepines have been used for cardioversion, but
     the dose required for amnesia varies greatly so they
     cannot be described as 'best'.
E   Benzodiazepines are anticonvulsants.

X.10   FFTFT

A,B,   Atropine, glycopyrronium and droperidol will, if anything,
D   reduce tone in the sphincter of Oddi.
C,E   Most opioids are said to increase the tone – morphine
        especially. Pethidine has less effect. The effect of fentanyl
        is not consistent, but the answer here is probably 'true'.

X.11   **FTFTF**

A   A pH of 6.9 is too low for an early sample: 7.1 perhaps.
B   There will be respiratory compensation for a metabolic acidosis.
C   The patient has normal lungs and is hyperventilating. The PaO_2 will be normal or high.
D,E   A standard bicarbonate of 11 mmol/l (compatible with the diagnosis) is a base excess of – 13 mmol/l.

X.12   **TTFFF**

C   The thoracic duct lies further posteriorly and is not related to the trachea.
D   The right recurrent laryngeal nerve has already looped under the right subclavian artery. The left recurrent runs under the aortic arch and then up between the trachea and oesophagus.
E   The phrenic nerves are more lateral.

X.13   **TTTTF**

A–C   The anatomy of the sympathetic chain in this region is variable; the stellate ganglion is only part of it. Block will extend from about C2 to T4.
E   The patient should breathe gently to help avoid pneumothorax.

X.14   **TTTTT**

C,E   The greater superficial petrosal nerve comes from the facial, and is eventually secretomotor to the lacrimal gland. This is not motor in the sense asked in **E**: motor means supplies muscle unless it is qualified, as in secretomotor.
D   The maxillary division lies anterosuperior in this approach.

X.15   **TTFTT**

A   In some patients the jugular vein may lie anterior to the carotid artery, but usually it is lateral.
C   The recurrent laryngeal nerves, not the vagi, lie between the trachea and oesophagus.

X.16   TFTFF

In a question giving laboratory findings, identify the abnormalities and attempt a provisional diagnosis from the stem before looking at the branches.

B,D   Urea is low in hepatic failure and when there is inappropriate ADH secretion.

E   A patient with a high bowel obstruction will lose gastric and duodenal secretions. Unless severely dehydrated they are unlikely to be acidotic, and would be hypokalaemic if anything.

X.17   TTTFF

D   In anterolateral infarction, there is ST elevation in leads I, aVL and V4–6.

E   ST elevation in leads I and aVR is anteroseptal. Posterior infarction is difficult: there are likely to be tall R waves in V1–2.

X.18   FFTTF

A,B,   None of these diagnoses explain the systolic and diastolic
E   murmurs.

C,D   The low diastolic pressure makes an aortic lesion more likely than a mitral lesion, although mitral valve disruption is probably more likely to cause the pulmonary symptoms and cardiac failure.

X.19   FFTT

VIPomas produce 'vasoactive intestinal peptide' and probably other active substances as well.

A   Hypokalaemia, if anything, as a result of the diarrhoea.

B   VIPomas do not cause steatorrhoea.

X.20   FTFFT

A,C,   A woman with hyperthyroidism will have a hyperdynamic
D   circulation (giving an increased pulse pressure), is likely to prefer cooler conditions and is more likely to have oligomenorrhoea than menorrhagia.

X.21   TFTTF

B,E   Addison's disease and tuberculosis cause poor appetite, debility and weight loss.

X.22   TTTFF

A   The citrate combines with Ca^{2+} ions.

C   Few of the platelets in stored blood are active after 24 hours; most will have formed aggregates.

E   *Hyper*kalaemia may occur, although the potassium is re-taken up by the red cells fairly quickly once warmed up within the circulation.

X.23   FFFFF

A   Horner's syndrome results from cervical sympathetic block. It does not alter the effects of noradrenaline.

B   A peripheral neuropathy affects peripheral vasodilation, which may be reversed by noradrenaline, but not abnormally so.

C   Noradrenaline has come back into fashion for treatment of low blood pressure in shock states. There is no suggestion that sepsis potentiates its effects.

D   The effects of noradrenaline are reduced by treatment with guanethidine (rarely given systemically now) because endogenous release is reduced.

E   Although extradural anaesthesia causes vasodilation, few would think of giving noradrenaline to support the blood pressure.

X.24   FTFTT

A   Potassium losses are increased after the trauma of operation.

C   Nitrogen losses are increased by catabolism and there is negative nitrogen balance.

D   The answer here is 'true', but it does depend on how much fluid is given.

X.25   TTFFF

C   Polycythaemia is uncommon in 'pink puffers', common in 'blue bloaters'. Many patients are not clearly in one or other category.

D   Pulmonary vessels are attenuated.

E   Cor pulmonale is infrequent, and usually terminal.

X.26   TFTTT

> **B**   Mydriasis (dilated pupils) rather than miosis (constricted pupils).
>
> **D**   The question implies simple acute primary hypoxia rather than hypoxia imposed on respiratory failure and a pre-existing hypercapnia. Hypoxia classically causes reflex tachycardia before bradycardia, though the tachycardia does not always occur.

X.27   TFFFF

> **B**   Vasodilators aid skin blood flow and can help trophic ulcers to heal, but they do not improve muscle blood flow.
>
> **C**   It is the cardiac and cerebral complications of arteriosclerosis that kill most patients.
>
> **D**   Many of these patients will have coronary vessel disease, but the symptoms may be masked by the inability to walk far.
>
> **E**   Pulse oximeters measure oxygen saturation, but do not measure blood flow effectively.

X.28   FTFTF

Laparotomy may be avoided by adequate investigations before taking the patient to theatre.

> **A**   Analgesia should be the first line treatment.
>
> **C**   Distension may be due to toxic gastric distension or paralytic ileus.
>
> **E**   Retroperitoneal haematomas are not necessarily an indication for operation.

X.29   TTFFF

> **C**   Respiratory arrest may be because of brain stem contusion or cerebral oedema: neither are indications for operation.
>
> **D**   CSF rhinorrhoea is not an indication for immediate operation.
>
> **E**   Fitting may be an indication for anticonvulsant therapy, but not for operation.

X.30   TFTTF

> **B**   Isoflurane is safe.
>
> **C,D**   These biochemical findings can be present in porphyria.
>
> **E**   Non-depolarising neuromuscular blocking drugs are safe.

Paper XI Questions

XI.1 **Suitable constituents of a cardioplegic solution for coronary artery bypass grafting include:**
A   potassium
B   bicarbonate
C   glucagon
D   magnesium
E   procaine.

XI.2 **In the management of ventricular fibrillation (VF):**
A   the initial treatment should be a DC shock of 200 joules
B   sodium bicarbonate 50 mmol should be given as soon as intravenous access has been gained
C   adrenaline 1 ml of 1:1000 is drug of choice for refractory VF
D   the maximum recommended DC shock is 500 joules
E   an antiarrhythmic agent should be given after three doses of adrenaline.

XI.3 **Techniques of topical anaesthesia suitable for nasal surgery include:**
A   Moffett's method
B   the use of cocaine paste
C   Krause's method
D   packing with 20% cocaine in adrenaline
E   Bodman's method.

XI.4 **Failure to maintain antihypertensive therapy up to the day of operation:**
A   causes intraoperative hypokalaemia
B   can cause severe postoperative hypertension
C   impairs renal function during surgery
D   causes exaggerated blood pressure responses to noxious stimuli
E   causes episodes of myocardial ischaemia during surgery.

XI.5   The laryngeal mask airway can be used safely to control the airway during:

A   hernia surgery
B   total hip replacement
C   emergency caesarean section
D   tonsillectomy in children
E   gastroscopy under general anaesthesia.

XI.6   Synchronised intermittent mandatory ventilation (SIMV):

A   is useful in neonatal resuscitation
B   is useful in weaning patients from artificial ventilation
C   is achieved by inducing rebreathing
D   reduces the risk of pulmonary barotrauma
E   fixes the patient's minute volume at a predetermined level.

XI.7   The following endotracheal tubes would be suitable for use in neurosurgical anaesthesia:

A   Oxford
B   Magill pattern orotracheal tube
C   flexometallic
D   Bryce-Smith
E   armoured orotracheal tube.

XI.8   To reduce the risk of acid regurgitation and aspiration in a patient presenting for caesarean section under general anaesthesia:

A   give an antacid preoperatively
B   give an H_2-antagonist preoperatively
C   apply cricoid pressure prior to and during tracheal intubation
D   induce vomiting preoperatively with apomorphine
E   extubate under deep anaesthesia with the patient in the left lateral position.

XI.9   The following are true of cystic fibrosis:

A   it is inherited as an autosomal dominant
B   it is one of the commonest inherited conditions
C   it is a condition specifically of the mucous glands of the respiratory tract
D   diagnosis can be confirmed by finding an increased sodium concentration in sweat
E   daily prophylactic antibiotics are a sensible precaution against chest infection.

XI.10 **Soda lime:**
  A contains 70% calcium hydroxide and 30% sodium hydroxide
  B may reach 60°C during active carbon dioxide absorption
  C humidifies the inspired gases
  D is contraindicated if sevoflurane is being used
  E provides about 1 h of absorbing capacity per 100 g.

XI.11 **Appropriate therapy for severe hypertension occurring after accidental ingestion of a tyramine-rich food by a patient on tranylcypromine includes:**
  A propranolol
  B phentolamine
  C moclobemide
  D guanethidine
  E chlorpromazine.

XI.12 **The Carlens double lumen endobronchial tube:**
  A is only suitable for intubation of the left main bronchus
  B has a carinal hook
  C was not originally designed for endobronchial anaesthesia
  D has its two lumens lying one in front of the other for extra rigidity
  E has a double endobronchial cuff.

XI.13 **The following are true of the anatomy of the large airways:**
  A the tracheal bifurcation is at the level of the fourth to sixth thoracic vertebra in the adult
  B the different angles of branching of the main bronchi are exaggerated in children
  C the right main bronchus is about 2.5 cm long in the adult
  D each lung normally has 10 bronchopulmonary segments
  E the right main bronchus is related to the azygos vein.

XI.14 **The diaphragm:**
  A takes its origin from the last six costal cartilages
  B is inserted into the first three lumbar vertebrae via the crura
  C from anterior to posterior is traversed by the oesophagus, inferior vena cava and aorta
  D moves 10 cm or more in deep inspiration
  E comes up to the level of the fifth rib in the mid-axillary line.

XI.15   The maxillary division of the trigeminal nerve subserves sensation from:
A   the skin over the temple
B   the bridge of the nose
C   the maxillary sinus
D   the upper teeth
E   the upper lip.

XI.16   The following are true of the recurrent laryngeal nerve:
A   the abductors are paralysed first in an organic palsy
B   unilateral palsies cause aphonia
C   the left nerve has a longer intrathoracic course than the right
D   stellate ganglion block causes temporary paralysis
E   bilateral paralysis is an absolute indication for tracheostomy.

XI.17   Hyponatraemia with total body depletion of sodium occurs in:
A   refractory heart failure
B   diabetic ketoacidosis
C   water intoxication
D   Addisonian crisis
E   renal failure.

XI.18   A 57-year-old man is admitted to hospital after a myocardial infarction. The ECG shows ST elevation in leads II, III and aVF, and ST depression in lead I. His blood pressure is 120/90 mmHg. Catheterisation shows a pulmonary artery pressure of 30/6 mmHg, a pulmonary 'wedge' pressure of 25 mmHg, a right atrial pressure of 8 cmH_2O, and a central venous pressure of 10 cmH_2O. The following are consistent with this clinical situation:
A   tricuspid regurgitation
B   left ventricular failure
C   left ventricular failure with fluid overload
D   simple fluid overload
E   right ventricular failure plus left ventricular failure.

XI.19   Acute cardiac tamponade is associated with:
A   massive ascites
B   increased 'a' waves on the jugular venous pressure wave
C   bradycardia
D   cyanosis
E   pulsus paradoxus.

XI.20   **In diabetes mellitus:**
A   insulin requirements decrease in pregnancy
B   renal papillary necrosis occurs
C   there is postural hypotension
D   serial glucose tolerance tests are used in assessing treatment
E   retinopathy is an early complication.

XI.21   **The following drugs have the recognised complication of causing convulsions:**
A   benzyl penicillin
B   halothane
C   primidone
D   insulin
E   cocaine.

XI.22   **Chronic constipation is a complication of:**
A   hyperthyroidism
B   hyperkalaemia
C   porphyria
D   hypercalcaemia
E   autonomic neuropathy.

XI.23   **The development of disseminated intravascular coagulation (DIC) is a recognised complication of:**
A   cardiac surgery
B   prostatic carcinoma
C   head injury
D   giving birth
E   haemophilia.

XI.24   **Typical anticholinergic effects include:**
A   dry mouth
B   increased gastrointestinal motility
C   bradycardia
D   increased sweating
E   bronchodilation.

XI.25   **The following are features of chronic renal failure:**
A   bleeding tendency
B   macrocytic anaemia
C   hypertension
D   splenomegaly
E   tetany.

XI.26   Prolonged cigarette smoking is associated with the development of:

A   laryngeal carcinoma
B   myocardial ischaemia
C   Buerger's disease
D   peptic ulceration
E   transitional cell carcinoma of the bladder.

XI.27   Pathological conditions which can cause cyanosis include:

A   polycythaemia
B   cor pulmonale
C   pulmonary consolidation
D   mitral stenosis
E   methaemoglobinaemia.

XI.28   Tumours of the salivary glands:

A   arise most commonly in the parotid gland
B   are most commonly pleomorphic adenomas
C   are usually malignant
D   when malignant tend to be radioresistant
E   should be biopsied before surgery.

XI.29   Cholangiocarcinoma:

A   is commoner in young women taking an oral contraceptive
B   presents with symptoms of obstructive jaundice
C   is associated with chronic ulcerative colitis
D   is associated with alcoholism
E   can be cured by a Whipple's operation.

XI.30   Complications of a Colles' fracture include:

A   wrist drop
B   median nerve damage
C   late rupture of tendons at the wrist
D   avascular necrosis of the radial fragment
E   frozen shoulder.

Paper XI Answers

XI.1 TTFTT

A Potassium (10–20 mmol/l) depolarises the myocardium and the heart arrests in diastole.

C Glucagon is an inotrope and therefore undesirable.

D Magnesium (16 mmol/l) reduces rhythmogenicity and protects against post-bypass damage caused by potassium.

E Procaine is a membrane stabiliser.

XI.2 FFTFT

Questions and answers on resuscitation in this text are based upon the 1992 European Resuscitation Council recommendations.

A First action is a precordial thump.

B Sodium bicarbonate is given later in the sequence.

C The guidelines state 1 mg, which is 1 ml of 1:1000 adrenaline.

D 360 joules.

XI.3 TTFFT

You are unlikely to know the details of all these techniques. Answer those that you are sure of, but leave other answers blank to avoid the risk of a negative mark: guessing is unlikely to help you.

A Moffett's method is a mixture of cocaine, bicarbonate and adrenaline.

C In Krause's method, the internal laryngeal nerves are anaesthetised in the pyriform fossae.

D The cocaine concentration is too high: 10% maximum.

E Bodman's method is lignocaine 1.25% solution with 0.5 ml adrenaline per 40 ml. Pour solution into each nostril with the patient's head hyperextended.

XI.4 FTFTT

A,C There is no reason why failing to give treatment for hypertension should cause hypokalaemia or affect renal function.

E This is difficult to answer with certainty, though it is true that hypertension *can cause* ischaemic changes in someone with *pre-existing* coronary artery disease. We have given the answer as 'true'; but the real truth is that there are many parts of anaesthetic (and medical) knowledge that MCQs do not test well (see Q VI.1).

XI.5   TTFTF

C   The laryngeal mask airway is useful for a failed intubation, but it does not prevent regurgitation and is not a safe technique, although it may be the best under certain circumstances.

E   How will the surgeon pass the gastroscope past the airway?

XI.6   FTFTF

C   There should be no rebreathing in an IMV circuit.

D   Mean intrathoracic pressures are lower and the patient will not 'fight' the ventilator.

E   The SIMV setting of a ventilator determines the minimum minute ventilation, but the patient's own efforts determine the actual minute volume.

XI.7   TFFFT

A   One of the earliest 'anatomical' tubes, designed specifically for head and neck surgery.

B   The Magill tube can kink and obstruct if the head is flexed.

C   Metallic tubes are used for laser surgery of the airway. They are expensive and offer no advantages in neurosurgery.

D   You would need detailed historical knowledge to answer this. The Bryce-Smith is a double-lumen endotracheal tube. This type of question is best left blank unless you *know* the answer. Guessing is as likely to lose you marks as to gain them.

E   An armoured orotracheal tube is the most common nowadays.

XI.8   TTTFT

D   Apomorphine-induced vomiting was advocated in the past. It is very unpleasant for the patient.

XI.9   FTFTT

A   Cystic fibrosis is an autosomal recessive. One in 25 Caucasians is a carrier.

B   True: the incidence is about one in 2000 live births.

C   It affects both mucus- and non-mucus-secreting glands throughout the body.

D   Sweat sodium is more than 70 mmol/l in affected children.

E   *Staph. aureus* infections are common in children, *Pseudomonas* infections in adults.

XI.10   FTTFT

A   Soda lime is 90–94% calcium hydroxide, 5% sodium hydroxide, 1% potassium hydroxide, plus indicators and silicates.

D   Sevoflurane decomposes slightly in soda lime, but this does not appear to be clinically important.

XI.11   TTFFT

Tranylcypromine is an 'irreversible' monoamine oxidase inhibitor.

C   Moclobemide is a reversible inhibitor of monoamine oxidase (RIMA). It may be better and safer as long-term treatment after the hypertensive crisis is treated, but is dangerous in the acute situation.

D   Guanethidine is an indirectly acting drug of slow onset, and is inappropriate.

E   Chlorpromazine is not perhaps the drug of choice for an anaesthetist, but it is recommended in the data sheet and is readily available to psychiatrists.

XI.12   TTTFF

A,C   The Carlens tube was designed for bronchopulmonary spirometry. The comparable right-sided tube is a White's.

D   The lumens are side by side, as in a Robertshaw (which is the most popular design).

E   One cuff is tracheal and the other endobronchial.

XI.13   TFTFT

A   The level of the tracheal bifurcation varies with posture and lung volume.

B   The angles of branching of the main bronchi are more equal in children.

D   The left lung normally has nine segments.

XI.14   TTFTT

B   The normal anatomy has insertion on the right into L1–3 and on the left into L1–2.

C   From anterior to posterior: inferior vena cava, oesophagus, aorta.

E   The fifth rib laterally is the same level as the eighth vertebral body posteriorly.

XI.15 TFTTT

B   The bridge of the nose is supplied by the frontal branch of the ophthalmic division.

XI.16 TFTTF

B   Unilateral palsies cause only hoarseness.

E   Tracheostomy may be needed, but few things are 'absolute'.

XI.17 FFFTT

A   There is sodium *retention* in heart failure.

B   A patient with diabetic ketoacidosis will be dehydrated and therefore hypernatraemic.

C   Total body sodium is diluted when there is water overload, but there is no net loss of sodium.

E   Though the answer here is 'true', not all renal failure is salt-losing.

XI.18 TTFFF

Look at the stem and think: probably an inferior infarct; not shocked; low pulmonary artery diastolic pressure and a high wedge pressure. The correct answers follow from this consideration. Incidentally, the clinical history and ECG findings are perhaps an indication for catheterisation but are irrelevant to the consideration of the results.

XI.19 FTFTT

A   There is no special association of acute tamponade and massive ascites.

C,D There will be *tachycardia* secondary to circulatory failure, which in turn causes cyanosis due to stagnant hypoxia.

XI.20   FTTFF

A   In pregnancy, insulin requirements *increase*; the renal *threshold* for *glucose* decreases.
D   Glucose tolerance tests are useful in diagnosis but not in the assessment of treatment.
E   Retinopathy occurs in juvenile-onset diabetics when they reach middle age.

XI.21   TFFTT

A   Penicillin causes convulsions in extreme overdose or if large doses are given intrathecally.
B   The myoclonus during recovery from volatile anaesthesia ('halothane shakes') is not convulsive activity.
C   Primidone is an *anti*convulsant with a structure similar to phenobarbitone.
D   Insulin causes hypoglycaemic convulsions (the now outdated 'insulin shock therapy').

XI.22   FFTTT

A   Hyperthyroidism causes *diarrhoea*.
B   *Hypo*kalaemia causes constipation.

XI.23   TFTTF

B   Some malignancies, for example bronchogenic carcinoma but not prostate, predispose to DIC. Abnormal fibrinolysis occurs with prostatic carcinoma.

XI.24   TFFFT

Typical anticholinergic effects include (**B**) *reduced* gastrointestinal motility, (**C**) *tachycardia* and (**D**) dry skin.

XI.25   TFTFF

A   Coagulation factors and platelet function are abnormal in chronic renal failure.
B   A normochromic, normocytic anaemia is likely.
E   Patients can be hypocalcaemic for a number of reasons in chronic renal failure but they do not get tetany. *Hyper*calcaemia is a *cause* of renal failure.

XI.26 **TTTFT**

C   Buerger's disease is also known as thromboangiitis obliterans.

D   Although the mortality from peptic ulcer is increased if patients smoke, the incidence of ulcer is not.

XI.27 **TTTTT**

Cyanosis is a clinical description referring to the blue colour of the patient. Usually it is caused by there being more than 5 g/dl desaturated haemoglobin in the blood, more uncommonly by methaemoglobinaemia or sulphaemoglobinaemia.

XI.28 **TTFTF**

B   The mixed parotid tumour is a pleomorphic adenoma.

C   The tumours are usually benign.

E   Salivary tumours can seed if biopsied or handled roughly at operation. Whether to biopsy depends on the site and likelihood of malignancy but should be done cautiously.

XI.29 **FTTFF**

A   Hepatomas have been described (rarely) in women on the pill.

E   Whipple's operation is for carcinoma of the head of pancreas. Cholangiocarcinoma is rarely resectable.

XI.30 **FTTFT**

A   The radial nerve carries no motor supply at this level and is unlikely to be damaged anyway.

D   Avascular necrosis is recognised after fractures of the scaphoid, not of the radius.

E   A common, early and incapacitating complication.

Paper XII   Questions

XII.1   **A 50-year-old woman presents for urgent surgery with acute dyspnoea caused by a huge goitre. She is clinically euthyroid and seems otherwise fit. Your management could include:**

A   a tracheostomy under local anaesthetic before surgery
B   carbimazole for 24 hours before surgery
C   a rapid sequence induction with cricoid pressure
D   the use of an armoured endotracheal tube
E   CT or MRI scan of the neck.

XII.2   **A 4-year-old boy is brought back to the operating theatre at 18:00 (6 pm) because he is bleeding after a tonsillectomy that morning. He is restless and obviously in some discomfort. His pulse is 145; his blood pressure is 85/60 mmHg. The following are true:**

A   he should be premedicated to calm him
B   the surgeon should secure initial haemostasis under local anaesthesia
C   anaesthesia should be induced with an inhalational agent
D   a nasogastric tube should be passed when he is anaesthetised
E   the risk of death from bleeding tonsil is negligible.

XII.3   **Suitable anaesthetic technique for correction of a squint in a 5-year-old child includes:**

A   the avoidance of intramuscular atropine
B   enflurane
C   intermittent positive pressure ventilation
D   tracheal intubation
E   retrobulbar block for postoperative pain relief.

XII.4   The following can delay recovery of consciousness after general anaesthesia:
  A   carbon dioxide narcosis
  B   peroperative use of narcotic analgesics
  C   residual neuromuscular blockade
  D   glycine toxicity
  E   mechanical hyperventilation.

XII.5   Conditions predisposing to adult respiratory distress include:
  A   severe abdominal sepsis
  B   renal failure
  C   massive intracerebral bleed
  D   prolonged, high concentration oxygen therapy
  E   extensive burns.

XII.6   Spread of local anaesthetic solution within the epidural space is influenced by:
  A   posture
  B   obesity
  C   pregnancy
  D   speed of injection
  E   age.

XII.7   The following are contraindicated in closed head injury:
  A   25 g mannitol intravenously
  B   homatropine eye drops
  C   diclofenac
  D   general anaesthesia with spontaneous breathing
  E   phenobarbitone.

XII.8   Indications for the use of lumbar epidural anaesthesia during labour include:
  A   placenta praevia
  B   pre-eclampsia
  C   prematurity
  D   cardiac valvular disease
  E   maternal exhaustion.

XII.9 **Conditions likely to be eased by sympathetic blockade include:**
A causalgia
B trigeminal neuralgia
C Raynaud's disease
D phantom limb pain
E pain associated with pancreatic carcinoma.

XII.10 **The action of mivacurium is enhanced by:**
A liver failure
B pseudocholinesterase deficiency
C gentamicin
D propranolol
E renal failure.

XII.11 **Appropriate treatment of a patient thought to have suffered an anaphylactic response to thiopentone would include:**
A intravenous hydrocortisone
B subcutaneous adrenaline
C volume expansion with saline
D isoflurane in oxygen
E intravenous chlorpheniramine.

XII.12 **A patient presents for left thoracotomy and resection of a large lung cyst. During anaesthesia:**
A nitrous oxide is contraindicated
B intermittent positive pressure ventilation should be avoided until the cyst is isolated from the bronchial tree
C halothane is a suitable anaesthetic
D endobronchial intubation is contraindicated
E topical endobronchial anaesthesia should not be used.

XII.13 **The following are true of the nerve supply to the arm:**
A the radial nerve supplies flexors of the wrist
B the radial nerve supplies skin on the opposing surfaces of the thumb and index finger
C the median nerve passes deep to the bicipital aponeurosis
D the radial nerve supplies skin over the back of the elbow
E the only motor fibres in the ulnar nerve are to small muscles in the hand.

XII.14   In the intercostal spaces:
A   the external intercostal muscle runs down and forwards
B   the nerves lie superficial to posterior intercostal arteries beneath the corresponding rib
C   the posterior intercostal arteries are branches of the internal mammary artery
D   about 3 ml of suitable local anaesthetic solution will block each nerve
E   the inner surface anteriorly is formed by the parietal pleura.

XII.15   The following are true of the nerve supply to the leg:
A   the upper inner aspect of the thigh is supplied by the ilioinguinal nerve
B   the upper inner aspect of the thigh is supplied by the genitofemoral nerve
C   the posterior division of the femoral nerve supplies the quadriceps muscle
D   the saphenous nerve is a terminal branch of the sciatic nerve
E   sensation from the knee joint is subserved mainly by the obturator nerve.

XII.16   Causes of a primary metabolic acidosis include:
A   vomiting
B   hydronephrosis
C   hypokalaemia
D   diabetes mellitus
E   intestinal fistulae.

XII.17   Causes of a hyperdynamic circulation include:
A   anaemia
B   myxoedema
C   pregnancy
D   Paget's disease
E   pulmonary embolism.

XII.18   A third heart sound:
A   is a normal occurrence in young people
B   occurs in left ventricular failure
C   occurs in mitral stenosis
D   occurs in constrictive pericarditis
E   occurs during systole.

XII.19 **The following conditions make the accidental intravenous injection of a small volume of air a particular hazard:**
A   ventricular septal defect
B   pulmonary stenosis
C   tricuspid regurgitation
D   patent ductus arteriosus
E   atrial septal defect.

XII.20 **In a patient with acute intermittent porphyria in whom a crisis is precipitated, associated symptoms include:**
A   coma
B   paralysis
C   skin lesions
D   tinnitus
E   mania.

XII.21 **Likely complications of ulcerative colitis include:**
A   anaemia
B   acute toxic colonic dilation
C   perforation
D   hypocalcaemia
E   hypoproteinaemia.

XII.22 **Portal hypertension occurs in:**
A   hepatic venous thrombosis
B   constrictive pericarditis
C   tricuspid regurgitation
D   ascending cholangitis
E   polycythaemia.

XII.23 **Reticulocytosis occurs in:**
A   acute leukaemia
B   treated vitamin B_{12} deficiency
C   haemolytic anaemia
D   sickle cell disease
E   thalassaemia.

XII.24 **Metoclopramide:**
A   is useful for opioid-induced nausea
B   is less effective if given after atropine
C   has only a peripheral action
D   has no extrapyramidal effects
E   can be given intravenously.

XII.25 On a chest radiograph:
  A the right hilum is higher than the left
  B Kerley B lines represent the superior pulmonary veins
  C the lesser fissure is on a level with the sixth rib in the axilla
  D a pneumothorax is best demonstrated on an inspiratory film
  E the carina is at T4.

XII.26 Clinical signs in a patient with chronic bronchitis suffering from acute respiratory failure include:
  A small volume pulse
  B cold extremities
  C elevated jugular venous pressure
  D tremor
  E papilloedema.

XII.27 Likely causes of surgical emphysema in a patient with vomiting, abdominal pain and dyspnoea include:
  A pulmonary infarction
  B pulmonary embolus
  C spontaneous pneumothorax
  D ruptured oesophagus
  E ruptured trachea.

XII.28 **Primary malignant tumours which commonly metastasise to the lung include:**
A   testicular seminoma
B   thyroid carcinoma
C   ovarian carcinoma
D   hypernephroma
E   breast carcinoma.

XII.29 **The following are true of carcinoma of the stomach:**
A   it is commoner in men
B   it is associated with achlorhydria
C   a longer history is associated with a better prognosis
D   to be curative the whole stomach must be removed at operation
E   palliative radiotherapy is useful.

XII.30 **Hypernephroma:**
A   is an adenocarcinoma
B   tends to spread via the venous system
C   presents most commonly as painless haematuria
D   is a cause of pyrexia of unknown origin
E   is a contraindication to intravenous urography.

Paper XII Answers

XII.1 FFFTT

A If the goitre is 'huge' the trachea will be inaccessible.
B Carbimazole is a treatment for thyrotoxicosis. The question states that this patient is euthyroid.
C Rapid sequence induction is hazardous when there is acute dyspnoea: you might fail to intubate the trachea *and* have difficulty ventilating by facemask. An 'awake' intubation is probably the wisest plan of action.
D Not the only possibility, but you certainly could use an armoured endotracheal tube.
E Thoracic inlet X-rays used to be requested. Scans, especially by MRI, are an excellent way of assessing the extent of the goitre and state and position of trachea.

XII.2 FFTTF

A,C These are arguable but, whatever is done, one must remember that the patient may be severely hypovolaemic. He should be resuscitated, *and* transfused if necessary, before induction (**E**).
B Using a local anaesthetic technique may be appropriate in an adult. It is certainly not appropriate in a 4-year-old.
D The stomach will be full of blood.
E Tonsillectomy is a common operation. It is regarded by doctors and patients alike as a minor procedure, but every year a few patients die.

XII.3 FTTTF

The question asks for a 'suitable' technique; it must be safe and sensible, but it may not be the way that you would give the anaesthetic.
A There is no need to avoid atropine, though it could be given intravenously at induction. The oculo-cardiac reflex should be blocked or attenuated in some way.
E Retrobulbar block might make the required degree of muscular correction difficult to judge.

XII.4 TTFTT

B A few patients are sensitive to remarkably small doses of opioids.

C Residual neuromuscular blockade does not affect *consciousness*.

D Absorption of glycine can cause many neurological symptoms and signs, including coma.

E This is arguable: does hyperventilation (in other words, hypocapnia) delay consciousness, rather than just delay the onset of spontaneous breathing? On balance it probably does delay consciousness.

XII.5 TFFTT

B Renal failure does not predispose to ARDS, though both may occur in severely ill patients.

C Some intracranial lesions cause reflex pulmonary oedema, and ARDS can follow massive transfusion. ARDS does not follow intracerebral bleeds.

XII.6 TFTTT

B Obesity affects the dose but doesn't affect the spread.

XII.7 FTFTF

A Mannitol reduces intracranial pressure by promoting an osmotic diuresis.

B Any drug that affects pupillary diameter hampers neurological evaluation.

C You could argue that both head injury and diclofenac cause peptic ulceration, but there is no published restriction on the use of diclofenac in head injury.

D Hypercapnia is likely if a patient breathes spontaneously, with the risk of cerebral vasodilation and increased intracranial pressure.

E Barbiturates go in and out of fashion as cerebral 'protectors'. Phenobarbitone is of more use as an anticonvulsant.

XII.8 FTTTT

A Placenta praevia is not a *contraindication* to an epidural, but it is not an *indication*.

D It was once held that cardiac disease was a contraindication to an epidural, but in general the reverse is now true.

XII.9   TFTTT

B   There is no sympathetic involvement in trigeminal neuralgia.

XII.10   TTTFT

A   The effective duration of block from mivacurium is three times longer in end-stage liver failure.

B   The duration of action of mivacurium is prolonged in pseudocholinesterase deficiency, though its effects are reversed by neostigmine once spontaneous recovery has started.

C   Gentamicin (as with all aminoglycosides) prolongs the action of all non-depolarising drugs – theoretically. This is a typical MCQ to which the answer is 'true' though in clinical practice at normal doses the effect is not obvious.

D   Catecholamines have effects on neuromuscular transmission in pharmacological experiments. These effects are not marked enough to affect the response to neuromuscular block in patients taking beta-blockers.

E   The block is prolonged about 1.5-fold in renal failure.

XII.11   TFTTT

B   Adrenaline is the mainstay of treatment for anaphylaxis. Subcutaneous adrenaline may be effective in mild anaphylaxis or if there is no intravenous access. Thiopentone reactions are usually severe, and there will be intravenous access. Intravenous adrenaline 0.1–1 mg repeated as necessary is more appropriate.

C   Volume expansion, either colloid or crystalloid, is important.

D   An inhalational agent may relieve severe bronchospasm, a cause of death in thiopentone anaphylaxis. Its effects as a peripheral vasodilator are unlikely to be important in a patient in shock.

XII.12   TTTFF

D   Endobronchial intubation may be needed.

E   There is no reason to avoid topical anaesthesia.

XII.13   FFTTF

A   Unopposed flexion causes wrist drop in a radial palsy.

B   The radial nerve supplies skin on the *back* of the hand.

E   The ulnar nerve supplies the long flexors as well.

XII.14 TTFTT

C The *anterior* intercostals (which anastomose with the posterior intercostals) arise from the internal mammary.
E The innermost intercostal muscle is the inner surface *posteriorly*, but the muscle ends at the anterior axillary line.

XII.15 TTTFF

A,B These are both true.
D The saphenous nerve is the terminal branch of the posterior division of the femoral nerve.
E The knee is supplied by the femoral, obturator and sciatic nerves: none is the *main* supply.

XII.16 FTFTT

A Vomiting causes a metabolic *alkalosis*.
C Hypokalaemia induces an intracellular acidosis and produces a metabolic alkalosis.

XII.17 TFTTF

B In myxoedema there is a low output state and reduced metabolic rate.
D Patients develop arteriovenous fistulae in the abnormal bone of Paget's disease.
E Cardiac output, if affected, is low in pulmonary embolus.

XII.18 TTFTF

C,E A third heart sound occurs during diastole and is associated with either tricuspid or mitral regurgitation.
D Constrictive pericarditis causes an early and high-pitched third sound, the 'pericardial knock'.

XII.19   TFFTT

The danger is an arterial embolus of air. Any right-to-left connection is a hazard even though, with normal haemodynamics, flow is from left to right through the defects.

XII.20   TTFFT

C   There are photosensitive skin lesions in some forms of porphyria but these lesions are not characteristic of an acute attack in intermittent porphyria.
D   Tinnitus sounds plausible but is not a typical feature.

XII.21   TTTFT

D   Calcium is not absorbed or secreted in the large bowel.

XII.22   TTTFT

C   Tricuspid regurgitation causes an extrahepatic, postsinusoidal portal hypertension.
D   Cholangitis affects the biliary tree, not the portal venous system.
E   Polycythaemia causes portal venous thrombosis and secondarily portal hypertension.

XII.23   FTTTF

Reticulocytosis indicates increased production of red cells. The count is reduced in acute leukaemia (**A**).
E   Thalassaemia is not a single entity and the blood findings vary according to the variety, but there is not reticulocytosis.

XII.24   TTFFT

B   Atropine counters the peripheral action of metoclopramide.
C   Metoclopramide causes central dopaminergic blockade which increases the vomiting threshold in the chemoreceptor trigger zone.
D   Extrapyramidal side-effects are especially likely in patients with renal failure, for unknown reasons.
E   Metoclopramide, but not prochlorperazine, is licensed for intravenous use.

XII.25   FFTFT

A   The left hilum is usually 1 cm higher than the right.
B   'B' lines are visible interlobular lymphatics. They are basal, horizontal lines seen when there is increased left atrial pressure.
D   Expiratory films are better for showing pneumothorax.

XII.26   FFFTT

The patient will be retaining carbon dioxide.
A,B   There will be vasodilation and a bounding pulse.
C   These patients are often oedematous because of sodium and bicarbonate retention without being in right heart failure. The wording of the question does not imply heart failure.
E   There is a rare association with hypercapnia of ventilatory failure.

XII.27   FFTTF

This is a poor question. How often does this combination of clinical signs arise? How often do you have to make a diagnosis with as little information as this? Is this a first presentation, or has the patient had an operation and *then* developed the emphysema? Or did the emphysema appear first? However, even with so many imponderables, you can still give sensible clinical answers.
A,B   Neither pulmonary infarction nor pulmonary embolism causes surgical emphysema.
C,D   Ruptured oesophagus must be the *most* likely cause; spontaneous pneumothorax could occur in a susceptible patient with abdominal problems.
E   Ruptured trachea is a rare injury, caused usually by violence or instrumentation. Connecting these signs by an isolated ruptured trachea is somewhat devious (other injuries in a road traffic accident?). This might be best answered 'don't know'.

XII.28 TTFTT

Note the word 'commonly'.

C   Ovarian carcinoma typically spreads transperitoneally.
Meig's syndrome is the association between a benign
ovarian tumour and a pleural effusion.

XII.29 TTTFF

C   This sounds paradoxical, but is so because the prognosis
depends on the histology.

D   The amount of stomach to be resected for cure (when
possible) depends on the site of the tumour (which
determines its lymphatic drainage).

E   Adenocarcinomas are resistant to radiotherapy.

XII.30 TTTTF

B   Tumour tends to grow into the renal veins.

E   Imaging is now more useful, but there is no
contraindication to intravenous urography.

Paper XIII Questions

XIII.1 After transection of the spinal cord above T5, factors likely to influence anaesthetic management of coincidental surgery within one month of the initial injury include:
A hyperexcitability of autonomic reflexes
B altered temperature regulation
C abnormal responses of skeletal muscles
D exaggerated baroreceptor response to intubation
E hypoglycaemia.

XIII.2 In the peroperative management of a patient presenting with severe hypertension caused by phaeochromocytoma:
A the first line of treatment is intravenous propranolol
B phentolamine should be used to stabilise blood pressure
C phenoxybenzamine is contraindicated because of its long half-life
D isoflurane may cause high output cardiac failure
E phenylephrine may be required after removal of the tumour.

XIII.3 Intraocular pressure is lowered by:
A hypocapnia
B isoflurane
C hypoxia
D morphine
E non-depolarising neuromuscular blocking drugs.

XIII.4 In a patient with a hiatus hernia, anaesthetic complications at induction may be reduced by:
A preoperative histamine H_2-antagonists
B preoperative antacid therapy
C preoxygenation
D topical anaesthesia of the larynx
E atropine premedication.

XIII.5 The following are effective methods of preventing stress ulceration in the critically ill patient:
A histamine H_2-receptor blockade
B sucralfate
C selective decontamination of the upper gastrointestinal tract
D magnesium sulphate
E nasogastric feeding.

XIII.6   Acute paracetamol poisoning is characterised by:
   A   increased plasma alkaline phosphatase
   B   encephalopathy
   C   hyperventilation
   D   increase in INR (prothrombin time)
   E   hypotension.

XIII.7   In closed head injury, the following are contraindicated:
   A   chlorpromazine
   B   clonazepam
   C   positive end-expiratory pressure (PEEP)
   D   elective intermittent positive pressure ventilation (IPPV)
   E   phenoperidine.

XIII.8   The following are absolute contraindications to epidural analgesia for an inguinal hernia repair:
   A   inadvertent dural puncture at the first space attempted
   B   ankylosing spondylitis
   C   multiple sclerosis
   D   allergy to local anaesthetics
   E   angina pectoris.

XIII.9   Epidural opioids:
   A   are only effective in high doses
   B   induce respiratory depression
   C   produce itching
   D   are contraindicated in thoracic surgery
   E   frequently produce hypotension.

XIII.10   **A depressed patient taking an irreversible monoamine oxidase (MAO) inhibiting drug such as tranylcypromine requires an elective anaesthetic. The following are true:**

A   the severe psychiatric problems of withdrawing the drug outweigh the anaesthetic risks
B   cardiovascular instability occurs in about 60% of patients
C   pethidine is the analgesic of choice
D   local anaesthesia is contraindicated
E   premedication with droperidol is recommended.

XIII.11   **The following statements about anaphylactic reactions to thiopentone are true:**

A   the incidence is one in 5000–7500
B   a specific antibody has not been identified
C   they are more likely to occur in atopic individuals
D   they are associated with classical pathway complement activation
E   IgE levels are unchanged.

XIII.12   **Adequate local anaesthesia for fibreoptic bronchoscopy in a 70 kg man requires:**

A   superior laryngeal nerve blockade
B   internal laryngeal nerve blockade
C   topical oral anaesthesia with amethocaine
D   at least 10 ml of 4% plain lignocaine
E   cricothyroid puncture.

XIII.13   **The following segments supply the movements or muscles:**

A   C5 and lateral rotation at the shoulder
B   C5–6 and flexion at the elbow
C   C6–7 supplies the long extensors and flexors of the wrist
D   C7–8 supplies pronation and supination of the forearm
E   T1 supplies all the intrinsic muscles of the hand via the ulnar nerve.

XIII.14   **The following are true of the spinal cord:**

A   the anterior spinal artery arises from the vertebral artery
B   the posterior spinal artery originates from the posterior inferior cerebellar artery
C   the anterior spinal artery runs in the anterior median fissure
D   fine touch and position sense are carried uncrossed in the posterior columns
E   the thoracic and lumbar lateral grey contains sympathetic neurones.

XIII.15   The following are true of the vagus nerve and its branches:
  A   it subserves sensation from the tympanic membrane
  B   it subserves sensation from part of the external auditory
      meatus
  C   the right recurrent laryngeal nerve hooks under the right
      subclavian artery
  D   the left recurrent laryngeal nerve hooks under the left
      innominate artery
  E   bilateral block at the base of the skull with a small
      volume of local anaesthetic gives good relief of the pain
      of mediastinitis.

**XIII.16   Specific inherited enzyme defects have been demonstrated
            in:**
  A   phenylketonuria
  B   cystic fibrosis
  C   favism
  D   adrenal hyperplasia
  E   malignant hyperpyrexia.

XIII.17   A profound bradycardia can be corrected by:
  A   applying pressure over the carotid sinus
  B   injecting a beta-adrenergic receptor blocking drug
  C   intravenous atropine
  D   intravenous isoprenaline
  E   eyeball pressure.

XIII.18   Causes of heart block include:
  A   aortic stenosis
  B   atrial myxoma
  C   congenital
  D   syphilis
  E   amitriptyline therapy.

XIII.19   Cardiac tamponade:
  A   occurs when more than 120 ml of fluid accumulates in
      the pericardial sac
  B   produces an increase in the central venous pressure
      accentuated in inspiration
  C   results in a radial pulse of small volume that fades in
      inspiration
  D   is unusual in viral pericarditis
  E   is better treated with diuretics than by needle aspiration
      of the pericardial sac.

XIII.20 Acute porphyria:
A is associated with abdominal pain
B is precipitated by barbiturates
C is diagnosed by the observation of port-wine stained urine
D occurs particularly commonly in West Indians
E is associated with sickle cell disease.

XIII.21 Cramping pain of the lower limbs occurs in:
A arteriosclerosis
B poliomyelitis
C central prolapse of an intervertebral disc
D thyrotoxicosis
E hyperparathyroidism.

XIII.22 The following are associated with ulcerative colitis:
A cirrhosis
B iritis
C psoriasis
D colonic carcinoma
E arthritis.

XIII.23 In a patient with progressive muscular dystrophy:
A tachycardia is a common clinical finding
B the myoneural junctions are not involved
C the myocardium may be involved
D thiopentone causes temporary peripheral paralysis
E inhalational anaesthesia is contraindicated.

XIII.24 Complications of immunosuppressive therapy with steroids include:
A hepatotoxicity
B hypersensitivity
C diabetes mellitus
D osteoporosis
E bone marrow suppression.

XIII.25   **An increased arterial partial pressure of carbon dioxide would be expected in:**
  A   pulmonary embolus
  B   diabetic coma
  C   vomiting due to uraemia
  D   gross obesity
  E   chronic bronchitis.

XIII.26   **Factors making postoperative segmental lung collapse more likely include:**
  A   recent upper respiratory tract infection
  B   cigarette smoking
  C   upper abdominal incision
  D   healed pulmonary tuberculosis
  E   allowing spontaneous ventilation peroperatively.

XIII.27   **Primary treatment of extensive full thickness burns should include:**
  A   50 ml fluid in the first 48 hours for each 1% surface area burned
  B   plasma in preference to plasma substitutes
  C   transfusion of whole blood
  D   measurement of arterial blood gases
  E   steroids.

XIII.28   **The following are true of hernias of the abdominal wall:**
  A   a strangulated femoral hernia is an indication for urgent surgery
  B   a strangulated inguinal hernia is an indication for urgent surgery
  C   direct inguinal hernias are always acquired
  D   a para-umbilical hernia never strangulates
  E   a Spigelian hernia presents as a mass in the iliac fossa.

XIII.29 **The following are perioperative complications of laparoscopic cholecystectomy:**
A   carbon dioxide embolism
B   pneumothorax
C   gastric distension
D   hepatorenal syndrome
E   sudden bradycardia.

XIII.30 **The following are true of carcinoma of the prostate gland:**
A   it is less likely in men who have had resection of a benign enlargement
B   it is the commonest origin of bony metastases in men
C   skeletal metastases are radiologically denser than normal bone
D   hormone therapy helps symptoms arising from both the primary and secondaries
E   orchidectomy is no longer part of the treatment of the disease.

Paper XIII Answers

XIII.1 TTTFF

C Suxamethonium can cause extreme hyperkalaemia.
D If the lesion is above T5, the cardiac sympathetics are denervated and baroreceptor responses are not exaggerated.
E Hypoglycaemia is not a feature.

XIII.2 FTFFT

A Alpha-receptor antagonists are required first; beta-blockade can cause cardiac failure and may increase blood pressure by antagonism of beta-mediated vasodilation in muscle.
C After initial control using the short-acting phentolamine, it is normal to convert the patients to the longer-acting phenoxybenzamine.
D High output cardiac failure will not occur if there is adequate beta-blockade.
E Sudden removal of vasoconstriction can cause sudden hypotension, for which phenylephrine can be used.

XIII.3 TTFTT

B Isoflurane reduces intraocular pressure by reducing blood pressure – unless carbon dioxide is allowed to increase.
C Hypoxia increases intraocular pressure.

XIII.4 TTFFF

C Preoxygenation is part of the technique of rapid sequence intravenous induction but does not in itself reduce the risk of regurgitation.
D Topical laryngeal anaesthesia removes the protective cough reflex; this may be combined with 'awake' intubation in the sitting position but, once again, without the rest of the technique it is not protective.

XIII.5 TTFTT

C Selective decontamination has enjoyed a vogue as a method of trying to reduce nosocomially acquired pulmonary infections. The evidence is contradictory, and at the time of writing not supportive, but selective decontamination certainly does not reduce stress ulceration.

XIII.6   TTFFT

    A   Liver function tests are a poor marker of the severity of poisoning.

    C   Hyperventilation only occurs late, secondary to hepatic failure.

    D   Clotting disorders occur because of liver damage.

    E   Hypotension is a bad prognostic sign.

XIII.7   FFTFF

    A   Chlorpromazine is sometimes used to control hyperpyrexia.

    B   Clonazepam is an anticonvulsant.

    C   There are some questions that are best left as 'don't know': this is probably 'true', because PEEP will increase intracranial pressure; but PEEP may be needed to improve oxygenation.

    D   Patients with head injury are often ventilated, though extreme hyperventilation is no longer thought necessary.

    E   Phenoperidine is a suitable drug if the patient is ventilated, although it masks pupillary signs. There have been occasional reports of phenoperidine increasing intracranial pressure, but at the moment it is not contraindicated.

XIII.8   FFFTF

    A   Standard practice would be to try again at a different space, insert a catheter and leave an epidural infusion of Hartmann's in place to try to prevent headache.

    B   Ankylosing spondylitis makes the injection difficult but is not a contraindication.

    C   It is impossible to prove that an epidural did not cause a relapse of multiple sclerosis, but it is not an *absolute* contraindication.

    D   Such allergy is very rare, but you would be foolish to proceed if the patient believed that he/she was allergic.

    E   This could generate much discussion – and is just the sort of topic that you must be prepared to discuss in a clinical viva.

XIII.9   FTTFF

    A   High doses make respiratory depression more likely and are unnecessary; low doses are usually effective.

    D   Epidural opioids can cause respiratory depression, but the risk must be balanced against the greater ease with which the patient can breathe when pain relief is effective.

    E   Sympathetic blockade will not occur unless the opioid is combined with a local anaesthetic.

XIII.10   FFFFF

A   If the surgery is elective the patient should probably be changed to moclobemide, which is a reversible inhibitor of monoamine oxidase (RIMA) (see Q XI.11).

B   Probably fewer than 10% of patients show cardiovascular instability.

C   Pethidine is the opioid most likely to cause hypertension; morphine or fentanyl is preferable.

D   Plain local anaesthetics are safe.

E   There is no recommendation for droperidol. It is not contraindicated, but do you ever use droperidol as a premedicant?

XIII.11   FTTFF

The treatment of anaphylaxis to thiopentone was asked in Q XII.11.

A   The incidence of anaphylactic reactions to thiopentone is more like one in 25 000.

B,D, They appear to be an IgE-mediated phenomenon not
E   involving complement. IgE concentrations are usually increased, although no specific antibody has yet been identified.

XIII.12   TTFFF

C   Though amethocaine lozenges are much beloved of older texts, the British National Formulary (BNF) states that amethocaine should *never* be used to produce anaesthesia for bronchoscopy.

D   10 ml of 4% lignocaine is 400 mg, which for plain lignocaine is an overdose.

E   Not required if the internal laryngeals are blocked in the piriform fossae, for instance using Krause's forceps.

XIII.13   TTTFF

D   Pronation and supination of the forearm is C6.

E   The intrinsic muscles of the hand are all T1, but are carried in the median nerve as well as the ulnar nerve.

XIII.14   TTTTT

A   The anterior spinal artery is the most important artery supplying the spinal cord.

XIII.15   TTTFF

   D   There is no innominate artery on the left: the left
        recurrent laryngeal nerve hooks under the aortic arch.
   E   Absolutely not!! Bilateral block would be exceedingly
        dangerous. Unilateral block of the glossopharyngeal
        nerve is sometimes used for glossopharyngeal neuralgia
        but there is inevitably spread to the other nearby nerves
        – look them up and work out what would happen with a
        bilateral block.

XIII.16   TFTTF

   B   Cystic fibrosis is transmitted as an autosomal recessive;
        the gene codes for a transmembranous protein.
   E   Malignant hyperpyrexia is not a disorder of an enzyme.

XIII.17   FFTTF

   A   This is a treatment for supraventricular *tachycardia*.
   B   Beta-blockers are also treatment for (some) tachycardias.
   C   Atropine will correct a tachycardia due to vagotonic
        stimuli. In other circumstances, blocking the vagus will
        alter autonomic balance in favour of a faster heart beat.
   E   This is a (rather hazardous) method of vagal stimulation.

XIII.18   TFTTT

   B   Atrial myxomas can impede blood flow, but are not
        associated with an electrical conductive block.
   E   Amitriptyline may cause heart block, particularly in
        overdose.

XIII.19   FFTTF

   A   The rate of development is more important, though
        probably upwards of 200 ml is needed to cause
        problems even if the effusion develops rapidly.
   B   Central venous pressure will be increased, but will still
        decrease on inspiration.
   C   So-called 'pulsus paradoxus' is an exaggeration of the
        normal. It is not pathognomonic of tamponade.
   E   Pericardiocentesis may be life-saving.

XIII.20   TTFFF

C   Although the urine may change colour, the diagnosis depends upon chemical testing for porphobilinogen in the urine.

D   Variegate porphyria is common in the Cape Dutch population of South Africa but not in those of black African ethnic origin.

E   There is no association between porphyria and sickle cell disease.

XIII.21   TTFFF

A,C   Intermittent claudication is a cramping pain; radicular pain is not cramping.

D   Cramping pain is not a feature of thyrotoxicosis.

E   *Hypo*parathyroidism and hypocalcaemia cause cramping (tetany).

XIII.22   FFFTT

A   Fatty degeneration and amyloidosis, but not cirrhosis, occur in ulcerative colitis.

B,C   Iritis and psoriasis have links with arthritis, but not with ulcerative colitis.

D   There is an 11% risk of carcinoma of the colon after 25 years.

E   The associations of ulcerative colitis are especially ankylosing spondylitis and sacro-iliitis.

XIII.23   TTTFF

D   Thiopentone is associated with exacerbation of familial periodic paralysis.

E   Volatile anaesthetics are not contraindicated, but must be used with care because of the possibility of ventilatory failure.

XIII.24   FFTTF

A,B,   Hepatotoxicity, hypersensitivity and bone marrow
E   suppression are not documented complications of steroid therapy, whether used for immunosuppression or for other indications.

XIII.25   FFFTT

A   Pulmonary embolus causes hyperventilation, and the $PaCO_2$ will decrease. This is a medical question. Don't make the mistake of thinking this question is asking what will happen when there is an intraoperative embolus in a ventilated patient, when the $PaCO_2$ *will* increase while the $PetCO_2$ decreases.

B   The $PaCO_2$ will decrease in compensation for the metabolic acidosis.

C   Although vomiting causes metabolic alkalosis, a uraemic patient would be acidotic and likely to have a low $PaCO_2$.

XIII.26   TTTFF

D   Healed tuberculosis is not normally a cause of acute pulmonary problems.

E   A common fallacy, especially among non-anaesthetists, is that artificial ventilation always makes postoperative pulmonary problems less likely.

XIII.27   FTFTF

A   For a 20% burn, this is 1000 ml: far too little, and fluid requirements are assessed 6-hourly, not for 48 h.

B,C   Plasma is always used in preference initially, though plasma substitutes are of course satisfactory if there is no plasma available. Blood may be needed later.

E   Steroids are not indicated unless there is direct burning of the respiratory tract.

XIII.28   TTTFT

A,B   The similarity of the wording is trying to suggest a difference between the two types of hernia. There are some – but a strangulated hernia at any site needs emergency surgery.

D   Umbilical hernias rarely contain bowel, but the contents can still strangulate and cause pain.

E   A Spigelian hernia passes upwards through the arcuate line into the lower part of the posterior rectus sheath. This is small print.

XIII.29   TTTFT

A,B   Carbon dioxide embolism and pneumothorax are
well-described complications.

C   Gas bubbles in the stomach, present preoperatively or
introduced during ventilation of the patient, will expand
if nitrous oxide is part of the anaesthetic and may
require aspiration through a nasogastric tube for the
surgeon to get a good view of the upper abdomen.

D   Hepatorenal syndrome is usually associated with severe
hepatocellular jaundice.

E   The porta hepatis is one of the areas of the body which,
when handled, may provoke a sudden severe
bradycardia.

XIII.30   FTTTF

A   The two conditions tend to occur in different parts of the
gland.

D,E   Orchidectomy is part of the available hormone therapy.

Paper XIV Questions

XIV.1 **A routine electrocardiogram from a 65-year-old man presenting for elective repair of a right inguinal hernia shows unifocal ectopic beats at a rate of 1:5 normal beats. Appropriate anaesthetic management would include:**
A   preoperative flecainide
B   lignocaine infusion commencing at induction
C   preoperative insertion of a transvenous, fixed-rate pacemaker
D   spinal anaesthesia
E   local infiltration during surgical repair.

XIV.2 **An anaesthetic technique suitable for septoplasty should include the use of:**
A   a throat pack
B   elective hypotension
C   nasal preparation with 10% cocaine
D   a non-kinking endotracheal tube
E   anticholinergic premedication.

XIV.3 **The following are indications for hyperbaric oxygen therapy:**
A   clostridial septicaemia
B   nitrogen narcosis
C   trophic ulcers of the ankle
D   carbon monoxide poisoning
E   decompression sickness ('the bends').

XIV.4 **Elective hyperventilation during anaesthesia for abdominal hysterectomy:**
A   reduces sympathetic tone
B   increases the MAC for enflurane
C   decreases cardiac output
D   reduces the risk of deep venous thrombosis
E   produces peripheral vasoconstriction.

XIV.5 If a patient remains comatose after successful cardiopulmonary resuscitation for ventricular fibrillation, treatment should include:

A   hypothermia
B   limitation of inspired oxygen concentration to 40%
C   corticosteroid therapy
D   doxapram
E   mannitol.

XIV.6 In a 4-year-old child with increased intracranial pressure, scheduled for insertion of a ventriculo-atrial shunt:

A   intravenous induction is better than inhalational induction
B   neuromuscular blockade is contraindicated
C   fluid therapy should be restricted to about 2 ml/kg/h
D   a cuffed endotracheal tube should be used
E   cardiac dysrhythmias are frequently seen.

XIV.7 A patient undergoing general anaesthesia for caesarean section should have her trachea intubated:

A   to ensure adequate fetal oxygenation before delivery
B   to prevent regurgitation of gastric contents
C   to ensure rapid deepening of anaesthesia
D   to allow bronchopulmonary lavage if necessary
E   because of an increased incidence of tracheomalacia in pregnancy.

XIV.8 Factors predisposing to the development of respiratory distress syndrome in neonates include:

A   prematurity
B   maternal diabetes
C   maternal pre-eclampsia
D   antepartum haemorrhage
E   fetal congenital heart disease.

XIV.9 **Immediate treatment of intra-arterial injection of thiopentone includes:**
A   intra-arterial heparin
B   procaine
C   phentolamine
D   sympathetic blockade
E   intra-arterial hyaluronidase.

XIV.10 **An abnormal response to suxamethonium can occur in patients suffering from:**
A   polyarteritis nodosa
B   dermatomyositis
C   systemic lupus erythematosus
D   dystrophia myotonica
E   hepatic failure.

XIV.11 **The following results suggest an acute exacerbation of underlying chronic obstructive airways disease with chronic bronchitis:**
A   a PaO_2 of 85 mmHg (11.2 kPa) on 24% oxygen
B   a $PaCO_2$ of 65 mmHg (8.5 kPa)
C   an actual bicarbonate of 22 mmol/l
D   a haemoglobin of 12.6 g/dl
E   a pH of 7.36.

XIV.12 **Considering the nerve supply to the larynx:**
A   sensation above the cords is via the internal branch of the superior laryngeal nerve
B   damage to the superior laryngeal nerve causes hoarseness
C   the internal branch of the superior laryngeal nerve pierces the aryepiglottic folds
D   the left recurrent laryngeal nerve is more readily damaged than the right
E   the recurrent laryngeal nerves supply all the intrinsic muscles.

XIV.13 **The femoral vein:**
A   lies behind the artery at first
B   lies medial to the artery at the inguinal ligament
C   receives the long and short saphenous veins
D   is valveless above its junction with the long saphenous vein
E   becomes the external iliac vein behind the inguinal ligament.

XIV.14   The ciliary ganglion:
    A   lies at the apex of the orbit
    B   must be blocked for cataract surgery under local
        anaesthesia
    C   carries parasympathetic fibres that relay and form the
        short ciliary nerves
    D   transmits sensory fibres without relay to the eyeball
    E   does not carry fibres subserving lacrimation.

XIV.15   Division of the sciatic nerve at the level of the ischial tuberosity causes:
    A   complete anaesthesia of the leg below the knee
    B   loss of the ankle jerk
    C   foot drop
    D   paralysis of the hip adductors
    E   paralysis of the rectus femoris.

XIV.16   The following are minimum daily requirements in the adult male:
    A   200 mmol sodium
    B   80 mmol potassium
    C   100 mg iron
    D   350 mg magnesium
    E   15 mg zinc.

XIV.17   Biochemical changes affecting the electrocardiogram include:
    A   hypokalaemia prolonging the P–R interval
    B   hyperkalaemia depressing the ST segment
    C   hyperkalaemia producing high peaked R waves
    D   hypocalcaemia prolonging the Q–T interval
    E   hypokalaemia producing tall U waves.

XIV.18   A pulse rate unchanged during and immediately after a Valsalva manoeuvre occurs in:
    A   aortic incompetence
    B   Horner's syndrome
    C   autonomic blockade
    D   diabetes mellitus
    E   heart failure.

XIV.19 In primary hyperparathyroidism:

A serum calcium is increased
B urinary calcium is decreased
C alkaline phosphatase is increased
D urinary phosphate excretion increases
E rarefaction of bone is visible on chest radiograph.

XIV.20 Severe diarrhoea is a complication of:

A diabetes mellitus
B guanethidine therapy
C hypercalcaemia
D hyperthyroidism
E carcinoid syndrome.

XIV.21 The following statements concerning diseases of the liver are true:

A jaundice due to monoamine oxidase inhibitors is cholestatic
B jaundice associated with halothane administration is more common in obese patients
C centrilobular hepatic necrosis is the classical histological picture seen in halothane hepatitis
D isoflurane maintains hepatic blood flow better than halothane during general anaesthesia
E anaesthetic management of a jaundiced patient should include intravenous mannitol.

XIV.22 Sickle-cell trait:

A is found in subjects homozygous for the HbS gene
B presents as severe anaemia
C is inherited as a mendelian dominant
D can be detected using the commercially available Sickledex™ test
E is a contraindication to the use of limb tourniquet.

XIV.23 Beta-adrenergic blockade:

A should be stopped 2 days before anaesthesia and surgery
B induces bronchospasm
C withdrawal may provoke hypertension and myocardial ischaemia
D produces irreversible bradycardia
E is contraindicated in conjunction with isoflurane.

XIV.24   **A metabolic alkalosis, persisting after elective partial gastrectomy despite adequate replacement of sodium chloride and water, is a strong indication of:**
   A   potassium deficiency
   B   low serum calcium
   C   low serum magnesium
   D   water intoxication
   E   intracellular sodium depletion.

XIV.25   **In a patient with obstructive airways disease of the 'blue bloater' type:**
   A   sputum is profuse and mucopurulent
   B   polycythaemia is uncommon
   C $PaCO_2$ is normal
   D   cor pulmonale is common
   E   alveolar gas transfer is normal.

XIV.26   **In fibrosing alveolitis:**
   A   the aetiology is frequently post-infective
   B   gas transfer is reduced
   C   hyperventilation occurs at rest
   D   the $PaCO_2$ is usually slightly increased
   E   chest radiography in severe cases shows pleural involvement.

XIV.27   **The following are of benefit in proven Gram-negative septicaemia:**
   A   cefotaxime
   B   metronidazole
   C   cloxacillin
   D   gentamicin
   E   benzylpenicillin with probenecid.

XIV.28   **Factors associated with anastomotic breakdown following colonic surgery include:**
   A   previous irradiation
   B   reversal of non-depolarising neuromuscular blockade
   C   intraoperative hypotension
   D   steroid therapy
   E   anaemia.

XIV.29   A Colles' fracture:

A   is a fracture of the lower end of the radius
B   results in forward and medial displacement of the distal fragment
C   is particularly likely in elderly women
D   is usually greenstick in a child
E   is a cause of frozen shoulder.

XIV.30   The following occur in dystrophia myotonica:

A   testicular atrophy
B   frontal baldness
C   optic atrophy
D   ptosis
E   diabetes mellitus.

Paper XIV   Answers

XIV.1   FFFTT

Enthusiasm for treating asymptomatic ectopic beats has dwindled.

D,E These options would be appropriate management whether or not ectopics were present; they are not the only reasonable anaesthetic techniques.

XIV.2   TFTTF

B Hypotension is not indicated for a septoplasty, although, when the patient is fit, it may make septorhinoplasty an easier surgical procedure.

E In the first edition the answer was 'true'; nowadays it is not regarded as obligatory. Nasal surgery has no direct cardiac effects although bradycardia may occur if the surgeon accidentally presses on the eyeball.

XIV.3   FFTTT

A Gas gangrene in the tissues can be treated by hyperbaric oxygen, but hyperbaric treatment will have little effect on septicaemia.

B,E Nitrogen narcosis develops in scuba divers breathing air at a pressure greater than 6 bar. Divers going below 50 m water depth require Heliox mixtures. Nitrogen narcosis is different from decompression sickness.

C Trials show that hyperbaric oxygen is effective treatment for trophic ulcers, but it is rarely used.

XIV.4   TFTFF

B The response to painful stimuli is modified by hypocapnia, which reduces the requirement for volatile agents.

D There is no evidence for any effect on thromboembolic risk.

E There may be less obvious vasodilation, but not peripheral vasoconstriction.

XIV.5   FFTFT

The implication is that the coma is caused by cerebral oedema.

A   Hypothermia is no longer recommended.

B   Appropriate inspired oxygen should be given to maintain saturation above 95%. If a pulse oximeter is not available, the highest possible concentration of oxygen should be given (see Q VIII.18, in which 28% inspired oxygen was the suggested limit).

D   Doxapram is a respiratory stimulant. It is an analeptic but does not reverse coma due to a cerebral insult.

E   Mannitol could be used with care: there could be a risk of fluid overload.

XIV.6   TFTFF

A,B   The aim is to prevent an increase in $PaCO_2$: intravenous induction and controlled ventilation.

D   Cuffed tubes are better avoided in young children.

E   Cardiac dysrhythmias are not a problem during insertion of ventriculo-atrial shunts.

XIV.7   FFFFF

Nobody in a country providing technically accomplished anaesthesia would dispute the stem of this question, but the reasons suggested for the statement are not valid.

A   Fetal oxygenation could perfectly well be achieved by giving the mother supplementary oxygen by any method; intubation is not required.

B   Intubation prevents *aspiration*.

C   Awareness is a problem especially of obstetric emergency anaesthesia, but intubation for rapid deepening is not part of the solution.

D   Intubation is needed for bronchopulmonary lavage – but why should it be necessary?

E   There is not an increased incidence of tracheomalacia in pregnancy.

XIV.8   TTTTF

E   There may be an association between congenital heart disease and respiratory distress but it is not known as an important predisposing factor.

XIV.9   TTTTF

The problem is best avoided! 2.5% thiopentone is less damaging than the original 5% preparation, but is still potentially harmful.

E   Hyaluronidase is injected subcutaneously.

XIV.10   TTTTT

A–C   All are associated with liver dysfunction, and thus possibly reduced plasma cholinesterase.

D,E   These are the more important branches to have marked correctly.

XIV.11   FTTFF

A   This PaO_2 is too high.

D   A chronically hypoxic patient would be polycythaemic.

E   The pH would be lower than this in an *acute* exacerbation. The usual pH could well be 7.36 or lower, a high bicarbonate compensating the increased $PaCO_2$.

XIV.12   TTFTF

B,E   The cricothyroid muscle is an intrinsic muscle although it lies outside the framework. Hoarseness is caused by loss of tension.

C   The internal branch of the superior laryngeal nerve pierces the thyrohyoid ligament and runs through the piriform fossa.

XIV.13   TTFFT

C   The short saphenous vein ends variably, but well distal to the femoral vein.

D   There are valves proximal to the sapheno-femoral junction: important to know for passing a catheter into the femoral vein.

XIV.14 TTTTT

C The parasympathetic fibres come via the oculomotor nerve, relay, and form the short ciliary nerves.
D Sensory fibres in the nasociliary branch of the ophthalmic division of the trigeminal travel without relay.
E Lacrimal secretomotor fibres follow a complex course from the facial nerve via the zygomatic branch of the maxillary division.

XIV.15 FTTFF

A The saphenous nerve, which is a branch of the *femoral* nerve, innervates the skin *down* to the medial malleolus.
D The adductors of the hip are innervated by the obturator and sciatic nerves.
E Rectus femoris is innervated by the femoral nerve.

XIV.16 FTFTT

A The daily requirement of sodium is 80 mmol, though in the short term (a few days) sodium conservation is efficient.
C One milligram of iron is lost each day, which needs an intake of 15 mg because of inefficiencies of absorption.
D,E These are not figures that one tends to remember (and don't guess!) but the levels of trace elements like zinc must be considered during prolonged intensive therapy. Magnesium is an important intracellular cation.

XIV.17 TFFTT

B *Hypo*kalaemia depresses the ST segment.
C Hyperkalaemia causes *high peaked T waves*, not peaked R waves.

XIV.18 FFTTT

A,E In heart failure there is a square wave change in blood pressure with no change in pulse rate. Aortic incompetence will not alter the pulse response unless there is also cardiac failure.
B The cervical sympathetics are not involved.
C,D Autonomic blockade or neuropathy caused by diabetes will impair the pulse response.

XIV.19   TTTTT

Parathormone specifically increases serum calcium concentrations by mobilising calcium from bone and by increasing calcium reabsorption and phosphate excretion in the kidney.

XIV.20   TTFTT

A   Diarrhoea occurs because of diabetic autonomic neuropathy.

B   Guanethidine was a useful second-line treatment for hypertension, but is rarely used now. It is still used, by injection, for pain of sympathetic origin.

C   Hypercalcaemia causes constipation, if anything. Diarrhoea causes malabsorption of calcium, and so itself causes *hypo*calcaemia.

XIV.21   FTFTT

A   Cholestatic jaundice occurs with phenothiazines, chlorpropamide and others. Monoamine oxidase inhibitors cause a hypersensitivity type of hepatitis (similar to halothane).

C   Centrilobular necrosis occurred with chloroform; halothane produces a hepatitic picture.

E   The osmotic diuresis caused by mannitol reduces the risk of hepatorenal syndrome.

XIV.22   FFFTT

A   The trait is the phenotype of the *heterozygote* genotype.

B   Sickle-cell *disease* presents as anaemia.

C   It is a mendelian *recessive*.

XIV.23   FTTFF

A,D When beta-blockers were first used, it was thought that myocardial depression under anaesthesia would be dangerous and the drugs were withdrawn before surgery. For many years now, it has been known that this is not true. They should be continued perioperatively. Their effects can be countered with infusions of direct-acting sympathomimetic drugs. Higher doses than normal may be needed, but the infusions are usually effective.

E   Of course not: but the drugs may act synergistically.

XIV.24 TTTFF

A–C All occur as a result of metabolic alkalosis, particularly if caused by prolonged loss of gastric secretions.

D Water intoxication is unlikely if saline has been given.

E Intracellular sodium depletion is possible but unlikely.

XIV.25 TFFTT

B,C Blue bloaters have raised $PaCO_2$ and are commonly polycythaemic.

XIV.26 FTTFF

A There are many precipitating causes, some of which are infective, but usually there is no known cause.

C Hyperventilation at rest is a sign of advanced disease.

D $PaCO_2$ increases as a terminal event.

XIV.27 TFFTF

B Metronidazole is effective against anaerobic organisms.

C,E Neither cloxacillin nor benzyl penicillin is effective against Gram-negative organisms.

XIV.28 TTTTT

A The large bowel does not have as good a blood supply as the small bowel and conditions for healing are more rigorous.

B Neostigmine causes contraction of the bowel and has been blamed by some surgeons for the breakdown of their handiwork. Whether the use of neostigmine really is a factor in anastomotic breakdown is not certain. Many things in medicine are not certain; it is inevitable that some will nonetheless be the subject of multiple choice questions.

XIV.29   TFTTT

A   The styloid process of the ulna may also be involved in a Colles' fracture.

B   The displacement described is a Smith's fracture, caused by a fall on to the back of the hand.

C   Postmenopausal women have osteoporotic bones.

E   Patients must be encouraged to move the arm to prevent the joints becoming stiff.

XIV.30   TTFFF

C   Cataract, not optic atrophy, occurs in dystrophia myotonica.

D   Ptosis is not a feature.

E   Cataracts occur in both dystrophia myotonica and diabetes, but diabetes is not a recognised association of dystrophia myotonica.

Paper XV Questions

XV.1 **The following are suitable premedication to allay anxiety in an extremely anxious patient undergoing carpal tunnel decompression as a day case:**
A temazepam 20 mg orally
B diazepam 10 mg intramuscularly
C diclofenac 100 mg rectally
D lorazepam 2 mg orally
E cinnarizine 30 mg orally.

XV.2 **A 69-year-old man is to undergo laryngectomy for a glottic tumour that is obstructing his breathing. He is taking beta-blockers for hypertension. He smokes 30 cigarettes a day. The following are true:**
A a preoperative chest X-ray is needed only if he has symptoms referable to the lower respiratory tract
B invasive monitoring of blood pressure is justifiable
C a subclavian central venous line will allow an air embolism to be aspirated
D a rapid sequence intravenous induction is a sensible approach
E the patient should be ventilated postoperatively.

XV.3 **Appropriate drugs for use during general anaesthesia for cataract extraction in an 80-year-old man include:**
A suxamethonium
B vecuronium
C promethazine
D enflurane
E hyoscine.

XV.4 **Oral intubation is extremely difficult in an emergency case and suxamethonium has already been given. A correct course of action is:**
A give more suxamethonium and continue to attempt oral intubation until successful
B hand-ventilate with a face mask while maintaining cricoid pressure
C perform emergency tracheostomy
D maintain cricoid pressure and place a laryngeal mask airway
E summon assistance and wait for resumption of normal spontaneous ventilation.

XV.5 **The following are true of Gram-negative septic shock:**
A vascular permeability increases
B tumour necrosis factor has been implicated
C the septicaemia may result from instrumentation of the biliary tree
D the fibrinolytic system is unaffected
E steroids should be given in the early stages to all patients.

XV.6 **Stellate ganglion block produces:**
A hoarseness
B ipsilateral mydriasis
C enophthalmos
D anaesthesia of the supraglottic larynx
E ptosis.

XV.7 **A patient has traumatic quadriplegia after an accident 1 week ago. Likely problems include:**
A intermittent positive-pressure ventilation causing hypotension
B adductor spasm of the legs
C increased resistance to suxamethonium
D hyperthermia
E bladder distension.

XV.8 **Contraindications to the use of lumbar epidural anaesthesia during labour include:**
A previous caesarean section
B fetal distress
C maternal haemorrhagic tendency
D unwilling patient
E maternal multiple sclerosis.

XV.9 **Potential complications of epidural infusions of opioid plus bupivacaine for postoperative analgesia include:**
A itching
B hypotension
C hypoventilation
D sedation
E urinary retention.

XV.10 **Thiopentone:**
A forms a precipitate if mixed with suxamethonium
B induces acute demyelination in patients with porphyria
C induces its own hepatic metabolism
D is an analgesic
E is the sulphur analogue of pentobarbitone.

XV.11   Antibiotics known to interfere with neuromuscular transmission include:
A   tobramycin
B   cefotaxime
C   gentamicin
D   amikacin
E   metronidazole.

XV.12   In a patient with bilateral bronchiectasis undergoing elective abdominal hysterectomy:
A   head-up should be avoided
B   endobronchial intubation is required
C   awake intubation is indicated
D   spontaneous ventilation with epidural anaesthesia is contraindicated
E   preoperative anaemia is a likely finding.

XV.13   The following are true of damage to the peripheral nerve supply to the arm:
A   tourniquet damage to the radial nerve causes loss of supination
B   traumatic damage to the ulnar nerve at the elbow results in a useless hand
C   damage to the median nerve at the wrist results in minor disability if the motor components are spared
D   fracture of the radial head damages the posterior interosseous branch of the radial nerve
E   a supracondylar fracture of the humerus can damage the median nerve.

XV.14   The following are true of the nerve supply to the anterior abdominal wall:
A   the skin over the xiphisternum is supplied by T7
B   the skin at the umbilicus is supplied by T10
C   the skin in the groin is supplied by T12
D   L1 divides into the ilioinguinal and iliohypogastric nerves
E   the ilioinguinal nerve supplies the skin over the anterior superior iliac spine.

XV.15   The sciatic nerve:
    A   contains the largest nerve fibres in the body
    B   supplies sensation to part of the back of the leg
    C   supplies sensation from the lateral side of the foot to the
         web between the first and second toes
    D   gives articular fibres to all the joints of the leg
    E   gives off no major muscular branches between 1–2 cm
         below the popliteal fossa and a line joining the malleoli.

XV.16   Acute intermittent porphyria presents as:
    A   acute chest pain
    B   haemoglobinuria
    C   intraoperative hypotension
    D   anaemia
    E   convulsions.

**XV.17   Likely clinical features in a patient with constrictive
           pericarditis include:**
    A   tiredness
    B   hepatomegaly
    C   a third heart sound
    D   a forceful apex beat
    E   pulsus paradoxus.

XV.18   When auscultating the heart, an opening snap:
    A   indicates a fixed rigid AV valve
    B   is louder during expiration
    C   occurs in mitral stenosis
    D   follows the second heart sound
    E   is best heard at the upper border of the sternum.

XV.19   Causes of systemic hypertension include:
    A   polycystic renal disease
    B   Cushing's syndrome
    C   myxoedema
    D   subarachnoid haemorrhage
    E   ischaemic heart disease.

**XV.20   The following conditions commonly increase the urinary
           excretion of 4-hydroxy, 3-methoxy mandelic acid (VMA):**
    A   malignant melanoma
    B   pregnancy
    C   phaeochromocytoma
    D   diabetes insipidus
    E   carcinomatosis.

XV.21 **Drugs used in the conservative management of ulcerative colitis include:**
A azathioprine
B indomethacin
C prednisolone
D codeine phosphate
E 5-amino salicylic acid.

XV.22 **Causes of cirrhosis include:**
A viral hepatitis
B haemochromatosis
C cardiomyopathy
D secondary syphilis
E cystic fibrosis.

XV.23 **Neurofibromatosis is associated with:**
A cystic bone lesions
B paraplegia
C phaeochromocytoma
D aortic coarctation
E albinism.

XV.24 **Dextran 70:**
A has an average molecular weight lower than albumin
B can cause acute anaphylaxis
C is largely cleared from the blood in 4 hours
D cannot be mixed with dextrose
E causes haemodilution.

XV.25 **The following are indications for renal dialysis:**
A serum potassium greater than 5 mmol/l
B plasma bicarbonate less than 10 mmol/l
C creatinine clearance less than 3 ml/min
D an increase in blood urea of 8 mmol/l/24h
E the onset of renal bone disease.

XV.26 **Pulmonary fibrosis occurs in:**
A hypersensitivity
B rheumatoid arthritis
C paraquat poisoning
D pulmonary embolism
E uraemia.

XV.27   Pulmonary oxygen toxicity is associated with:
- A   ventilation on the intensive care unit at an $Fi\ O_2$ of 0.8 for 48 h
- B   breathing air at extreme altitude
- C   increased metabolic rate
- D   2.5 bar oxygen in a hyperbaric chamber
- E   anaemia.

XV.28   A 27-year-old woman with a hydronephrosis undergoes an uncomplicated ureteroscopy and stone removal. She develops a temperature of 39.6°C shortly afterwards in the recovery ward. The following are likely causes:
- A   bacteraemia
- B   postoperative chest infection
- C   malignant hyperpyrexia
- D   pulmonary embolus
- E   halothane shakes.

XV.29   The following are true of diverticulitis:
- A   the rectum is commonly affected
- B   the incidence increases with age
- C   there is an increased risk of malignant change
- D   an acute attack should be diagnosed by a barium enema
- E   a low residue diet is recommended for patients with chronic symptoms.

XV.30   The following are true of Paget's disease of bone:
- A   it is a rare disease
- B   it is a disease of long bones
- C   pathological fractures occur
- D   sarcomatous change is likely in long-standing disease
- E   surgery, if needed, is easy.

Paper XV Answers

XV.1 TFFFF

B Intramuscular diazepam is a painful injection, and absorption is unpredictable.

C Diclofenac is useful for postoperative pain, but is unlikely to reassure the patient!

D Lorazepam is an excellent anxiolytic, but produces prolonged amnesia, which is undesirable if early discharge is required.

E Cinnarizine is an antiemetic, but not an anxiolytic.

XV.2 FTFFF

A He *should* have a chest X-ray: he may have a coexisting inoperable bronchogenic carcinoma.

C A central line may help in the rare event of gas embolism, but the subclavian approach will restrict surgical access, particularly if a skin flap needs to be swung. A long line from the arm would be better – and there is a better indication than air embolism: to monitor cardiac filling.

D Induction in ventilatory obstruction is a much-asked question. There are a number of approaches, but this is not one.

E There is no indication here for postoperative ventilation.

XV.3 TTTTF

You can assume that a local technique is for some reason not appropriate: this is not a trick to which the answer is 'General anaesthesia is not indicated at all'. All these drugs (except hyoscine) are reasonable drugs to use, even if they are not your choice.

E Hyoscine can cause serious confusion in the elderly.

XV.4 FTFTT

A More suxamethonium and repeated attempts to place a tracheal tube is the ideal recipe for cerebral hypoxia.

C Emergency tracheostomy is the last resort for failure to *ventilate*, not failure to *intubate*. In any case, cricothyroid puncture is quicker and complications are less likely.

D This has been described although cricoid pressure makes correct placement of the mask difficult and the laryngeal mask airway does not prevent regurgitation.

XV.5   TTTFF

    D   Fibrinolytic activation is responsible for many of the bleeding problems that occur in this condition.

    E   There was a vogue for steroids in the 1980s, but they are not currently recommended. They either have no effect or worsen outcome.

XV.6   FFTFT

    A   There will be hoarseness only if the local anaesthetic spreads to block the recurrent laryngeal nerve.

    B   Stellate block constricts the pupil (miosis).

    D   This is the superior laryngeal nerve.

XV.7   TTFFT

This is acute section of the spinal cord, with interruption of the sympathetic supply.

    C   The patient should not be given suxamethonium because of potassium release but there is no change in sensitivity to the drug.

    D   Vasodilation will cause cooling and hypothermia.

XV.8   FFTTF

    B   Epidurals are often used to facilitate assisted delivery.

    D   Patients must not, with a few exceptions, be given treatment against their will.

    E   There is no evidence that epidurals cause relapse of multiple sclerosis. Nonetheless, many anaesthetists are wary and will think the answer 'true'.

XV.9   TTTTT

    A,B,   are common; **C** and **D** are less common but potentially

    E   more serious.

XV.10   TTFFT

    C   Although some barbiturates are specific enzyme inducers, thiopentone is not long-acting enough to do this.

    D   Thiopentone has no analgesic properties.

XV.11   TFTTF

A,C,   A common MCQ but a rare clinical problem
D   (see Q XII.10).
B,E   Neither has been implicated.

XV.12   TFFFT

A   Head-down permits lung drainage.
B   Endobronchial intubation is not necessary for an
       abdominal procedure. There is no need to isolate the
       lungs from one another.
C   Awake intubation is not necessary.
D   Spontaneous breathing is probably not the technique of
       choice as coughing may be a problem but, combined
       with an epidural, is not contraindicated.

XV.13   FFFTT

A   Tourniquet damage to the radial nerve is in the upper
       arm. Supination in flexion is biceps (supplied by the
       musculocutaneous nerve).
B   Trick movements compensate for the loss of the muscles
       supplied by the ulnar nerve.
C   Loss of the palmar sensation subserved by the median
       nerve is a major disability.
D   The posterior interosseous branch of the radial nerve is
       a motor branch.

XV.14   TTFTF

C   The groin is innervated by L1.
E   The ilioinguinal nerve does not supply the skin of the
       anterior abdominal wall. It passes through the inguinal
       ring to supply skin over the inner thigh and part of the
       genitalia.

XV.15 FTFTF

A   The sciatic is the largest peripheral nerve in the body, but its fibres have the same range of diameters as any other mixed nerve.

C   Its branches supply the entire foot except for a variable area between the medial malleolus and the base of the great toe (the area supplied by the saphenous from the femoral nerve).

E   This sounds very impressive, but the sciatic nerve terminates above the popliteal fossa where it divides into the tibial and common peroneal nerves.

XV.16 FFFFT

A   Acute intermittent porphyria presents as acute *abdominal* pain.

B   The abnormal porphyrins, not haemoglobin, colour the urine.

C   There may be *hyper*tension.

D   Porphyria does not usually cause anaemia.

XV.17 TTTFT

D   The apex beat will be remote and hard to feel.

E   There is pulsus paradoxus, with a rapid, low-volume pulse.

XV.18 FTTTF

A   An opening snap means a mobile, not a fixed, valve.

E   It is best heard just inside the apex of the heart.

XV.19 TTFTF

C   There may be *hypo*tension in myxoedema.

D   Hypertension is both a causative factor in subarachnoid haemorrhage and a clinical sign after a bleed.

E   Ischaemic heart disease is associated with hypertension but is not a cause.

XV.20 FFTFF

A,B,   VMAs are metabolites of catecholamines and their
D,E   urinary excretion is not *commonly* increased in these conditions.

XV.21 TFTTT

B   Indomethacin is a non-steroidal anti-inflammatory drug that tends to *cause* bowel ulceration.

XV.22 TTTFT

D   Congenital, but not secondary, syphilis causes cirrhosis.

XV.23 TTTTF

A   Cystic bone lesions are secondary to skeletal abnormalities or caused by expanding neurofibromas in the spinal cord.

C   Of patients with von Recklinghausen's disease, 1% develop phaeochromocytomas. Of patients presenting with phaeochromocytomas, 15% have von Recklinghausen's disease.

E   Albinism is a separate condition of abnormal pigmentation. Increased freckling and café-au-lait spots occur in neurofibromatosis.

XV.24 FTFFT

A   The molecular weight of albumin is 67 000.

C   Dextran's biological half-life is about 12–16 h.

D   Dextran 70 is a solution in 5% dextrose or 0.9% saline.

XV.25 FTFTF

A,B When considering whether to start dialysis the rate of change matters more than the absolute measurements, but in established renal failure 6–7 mmol/l potassium or 10–15 mmol/l bicarbonate are indications for dialysis.

E   Bone disease is not a consideration.

XV.26 TTTTT

A   Examples are farmer's lung and bird-fancier's lung.

D   Fibrosis is a late complication of those pulmonary emboli that cause multiple pulmonary infarcts.

XV.27   TFFFF

A   Chronic oxygen toxicity develops insidiously. Inspired oxygen of 80% causes toxicity in some patients.

B   Extreme altitude has its problems, but oxygen toxicity is not one of them. Oxygen partial pressures are decreased, not increased, at altitude.

C,E Oxygen toxicity is a direct effect of oxygen on the lungs.

D   Acute oxygen toxicity (within minutes) can occur in hyperbaric chambers. Oxygen at very high inspired partial pressure causes convulsions but has no acute effect on the lung parenchyma.

XV.28   TFTFF

A   Bacteraemia can occur if the hydronephrosis was infected.

B,D In the recovery ward is too early postoperatively to develop a chest infection. Pulmonary embolus is extremely unlikely (and does not cause an early pyrexia).

C   Malignant hyperpyrexia is a rare condition – but more likely than an embolus in the early postoperative period. It must be considered.

E   Severe shaking can occur but does not cause pyrexia.

XV.29   FTFFF

A   The rectum is not affected by diverticular disease.

C   Diverticular disease is not premalignant. However, it is important not to miss a coexisting cancer.

D   A barium enema may cause perforation.

E   *Bulking* agents are prescribed.

XV.30   FFTFF

A,D These branches allow some discussion of what 'rare' and 'likely' mean. It is not possible to define absolute figures, but one in 20 of the population will have Paget's disease (though only about 10% of them will have important symptoms) by the age of 75. That is not 'rare'. Sarcomas occur in about 2% of sufferers. Whether that is 'rare' is arguable, but it is certainly not 'likely'.

B   The disease is most obvious in the long bones, but any bone can be affected.

E   Surgery is difficult and hazardous because the bone is very hard and abnormally vascular because of arteriovenous shunts in the bone.

Paper XVI Questions

XVI.1 **Trismus is a recognised presentation of:**
A   pericoronitis
B   quinsy
C   fractured jaw
D   submandibular salivary gland stone
E   Hodgkin's lymphoma.

XVI.2 **Cardiac output can be measured in the clinical situation by:**
A   transthoracic impedance measurements
B   thermodilution techniques
C   ballistocardiography
D   Doppler ultrasound
E   thallium scanning.

XVI.3 **The following provide reliable measures of the depth of anaesthesia:**
A   auditory evoked potentials
B   sensory evoked potentials
C   cerebral function monitors
D   the Maddox wing
E   the isolated forearm technique.

XVI.4 **Carbon dioxide production is:**
A   reduced by halothane anaesthesia
B   increased by parenteral nutrition
C   increased during convulsions
D   increased by acetazolamide
E   increased by mechanical hyperventilation.

XVI.5 **Intermittent positive pressure ventilation (IPPV) is likely to be needed postoperatively if a patient:**
A   has a postoperative arterial PCO_2 of 80 mmHg (10.7 kPa)
B   has a postoperative arterial PO_2 of 60 mmHg (8.0 kPa)
C   has pain on coughing
D   has a preoperative vital capacity of 2 litres
E   has a preoperative FEV_1/FVC of 30%.

XVI.6   **In an unconscious patient, thought to be suffering from a ruptured intracranial aneurysm, anaesthesia for carotid angiography:**
A   should include hyperventilation
B   should avoid inhalational agents
C   should commence with a 'rapid sequence' induction
D   should include elective induced hypotension
E   should be preceded by injection of an intravenous anticholinergic drug.

XVI.7   **Relaxation of the pregnant uterus is produced by:**
A   epidural anaesthesia
B   nitrous oxide
C   ritodrine
D   halothane
E   amyl nitrate.

XVI.8   **The following are true of the Ayre's T-piece breathing system:**
A   the internal diameter of the reservoir tube should be 1 cm
B   it behaves similarly to a Bain system
C   the reservoir tube is of sufficient capacity to prevent rebreathing
D   the fresh gas flow for a child of 6 months breathing spontaneously should be 5 l/min
E   fresh gas flow should be at least twice the patient's minute volume during spontaneous ventilation.

XVI.9   **The following are true of anaesthetic vapours:**
A   MAC increases in pyrexial patients
B   MAC alters with age
C   patients breathing isoflurane should be given no more than 20 ml of local anaesthetic solution containing 1:200 000 adrenaline
D   desflurane is not a trigger of malignant hyperpyrexia
E   desflurane is suitable for gaseous induction of anaesthesia in children.

XVI.10   **The following cause pupillary dilation:**
A   intravenous neostigmine
B   intravenous trimetaphan
C   intravenous naloxone
D   sodium nitroprusside
E   intramuscular atropine.

XVI.11   A left-sided Robertshaw double lumen endobronchial tube:
A   is suitable for left lower lobectomy
B   is suitable for a right-sided bronchopleural fistula
C   has its two lumens side by side
D   is better than a right-sided tube if there is a choice
E   is contraindicated in a patient with a right pneumothorax.

XVI.12   The following are true of the brachial plexus:
A   it forms from the anterior primary rami of C1–T5
B   the lateral cord has contributions from C5–7
C   the posterior cord has contributions from C5–T1
D   the three cords are related to the first rib
E   the median nerve is the continuation of the medial cord.

XVI.13   The following are important to the competence of the normal oesophago-gastric junction:
A   a sling of diaphragmatic smooth muscle
B   folds of mucosa
C   intra-abdominal pressure compressing the oesophageal lumen
D   head-up position
E   keeping airway pressure less than 30 cmH$_2$O during mechanical ventilation.

XVI.14   The mandibular division of the trigeminal nerve:
A   leaves the cranium through the foramen spinosum
B   can be blocked by slipping anteriorly off the lateral pterygoid plate
C   has no motor fibres
D   supplies sensation to the inside and outside of the cheek
E   supplies sensation to the skin of the temple.

XVI.15   Bilateral damage to the recurrent laryngeal nerves:
A   causes aphonia
B   causes respiratory embarrassment
C   causes tetany
D   prevents the normal inspiratory abduction of the cords
E   allows the vocal cords to assume the cadaveric position.

XVI.16   Abnormally high plasma potassium causes:
A   U waves on the electrocardiogram
B   increased amplitude of the P waves
C   prolonged QRS complexes
D   ventricular fibrillation
E   increased digitalis toxicity.

XVI.17   Common complications of acute myocardial infarction include:
A   hypertension
B   left ventricular failure
C   ventriculo-septal defect
D   ventricular aneurysm
E   sinus bradycardia.

XVI.18   The T wave of the ECG:
A   is repolarisation of the ventricles
B   is about 0.5 mV in the standard leads
C   decreases in amplitude in hypokalaemia
D   increases in amplitude in digitalis toxicity
E   is normal in atrial fibrillation.

XVI.19   The following are true of adult panhypopituitarism:
A   its eponym is Sheehan's disease
B   there is hypoglycaemia
C   there is adrenal insufficiency
D   there is amenorrhoea
E   treatment includes mineralocorticoids.

XVI.20   Syncope occurs:
A   in diabetes mellitus
B   in aortic stenosis
C   in haemophilia
D   after a bout of coughing
E   when standing for long periods in hot weather.

XVI.21   Likely causes of persistent diarrhoea include:
A   thyrotoxicosis
B   intestinal intussusception
C   Crohn's disease
D   foreign travel
E   hypokalaemia.

XVI.22 Primary haemostasis depends upon:

A blood coagulation
B platelet aggregation and adhesiveness
C vascular factors
D prostaglandin release
E serotonin.

XVI.23 Myasthenic (Eaton–Lambert) syndrome differs from myasthenia gravis in that:

A there is normal sensitivity to depolarising neuromuscular blocking drugs in myasthenic syndrome
B the electromyograph is of decreased amplitude in myasthenic syndrome
C there is greater sensitivity to non-depolarising neuromuscular blocking drugs in myasthenic syndrome
D the weakness in myasthenic syndrome improves if the muscles are stimulated repetitively
E guanethidine reduces muscular weakness in patients with myasthenic syndrome.

XVI.24 In aspirin overdose:

A coma is common
B the patient may complain of tinnitus
C forced acid diuresis should be considered if the plasma salicylate exceeds 600 mg/l (4.3 mmol/l)
D hyperventilation is usual
E acidosis is usual.

XVI.25 In pulmonary embolism:

A serum lactic dehydrogenase concentrations are raised
B the characteristic ECG changes are S1, Q3, T3
C warfarin is a suitable first-line anticoagulant
D high dose steroids are indicated
E the chest X-ray appearance is characteristic.

XVI.26 Bilateral hilar lymphadenopathy is a diagnostic feature of:

A pulmonary tuberculosis
B Hodgkin's disease
C sarcoidosis
D pneumoconiosis
E systemic lupus erythematosus (SLE).

XVI.27 Acute pancreatitis causes:

A disseminated intravascular coagulation
B paralytic ileus
C hypocalcaemia
D hypoxia
E hyperkalaemia.

XVI.28 The early symptoms and signs of acute arterial occlusion of the lower limb are:

A pain
B paralysis
C pallor
D oedema
E a cold foot.

XVI.29 When a gallstone impacts in a bile duct:

A the gallbladder is easily palpable
B there is jaundice before pain
C the urine becomes dark
D an urgent cholecystectomy is essential
E liver function rapidly becomes depressed.

XVI.30 The following are true of rupture of the bladder:

A most cases are secondary to acute urinary retention
B there is a painful desire to pass urine
C intravenous pyelography is a useful investigation
D a small urethral catheter should be passed before surgery
E the need for surgery is urgent.

Paper XVI Answers

XVI.1 TTTFF
  C   Trismus is especially likely if there is fracture of the ramus.
  D   A stone in the submandibular gland presents with local swelling and difficulty swallowing, but not with trismus.
  E   Lymphoma may present with facial swellings, but trismus is not a typical feature.

XVI.2 TTFTF
  C   This research technique has been used for measuring cardiac output but is not practical clinically.
  E   Thallium scanning is for assessing ventricular performance, not cardiac output.

XVI.3 FFFFF
  Unfortunately none of these is reliable, though each has particular uses.
  D   The Maddox wing is used to assess recovery from anaesthesia, not the depth of anaesthesia.

XVI.4 TTTFF
  D   Acetazolamide does not affect carbon dioxide production, but slows its conversion to carbonic acid.
  E   Carbon dioxide *output* is increased when hyperventilation is started, but production is not affected. If mechanical ventilation is indicated to relieve the effort of breathing in ventilatory failure, then carbon dioxide production will *decrease*.

XVI.5 TFFFF
  Note the word 'likely'.
  B   IPPV is not indicated if the hypoxia is a single isolated finding. Increased inspired oxygen is the first-line treatment.
  C–E None of these is an indication for elective postoperative ventilation, although they do indicate that good postoperative analgesia will be necessary to prevent further deterioration.

XVI.6 **TFTFT**

A,B Controlled ventilation decreases the $PaCO_2$, causing vasoconstriction, which improves the image. There is no problem with inhalational agents used with controlled ventilation.

D Induced hypotension may severely reduce cerebral blood flow.

E An anticholinergic drug should be given because of the likelihood of carotid sinus stimulation.

XVI.7 **FFTTT**

A Epidural anaesthesia may reduce discoordinate uterine contractions but does not relax the uterus.

C Ritodrine is a beta-sympathomimetic drug used to prevent premature labour.

D Halothane (and other inhalational agents) relaxes uterine muscle. High concentrations should be avoided during caesarean section under general anaesthesia.

E Nitrates relax the uterus. Amyl nitrate was used to relax the uterus to hasten delivery of a second twin, but is no longer in the BNF. It is a recreational drug of abuse.

XVI.8 **TTFTT**

The figures for fresh gas flow are the ones generally quoted. In practice, capnography may permit considerably lower flows.

C The reservoir tube prevents dilution of inspired gas by room air, not rebreathing of exhaled gases.

XVI.9 **TTFFF**

B MAC peaks at 1–6 months and decreases thereafter.

C Up to 50 ml of 1:200 000 adrenaline is safe (but may be more than the permitted dose of the local anaesthetic).

E Desflurane commonly causes coughing, breath-holding and salivation.

XVI.10 **FTFFF**

A The pupillary dilation that occurs in clinical practice after an injection of neostigmine is caused by the general process of reversal of anaesthesia and arousal of the patient. Normal doses of intravenous atropine have no more effect than intramuscular **(E)**.

C Naloxone will reverse pupillary constriction only if opioid-induced.

D Nitroprusside has no effect on the pupil.

E Intramuscular atropine in normal dosage has little, if any, effect.

XVI.11   TTTTF

A   The tube goes no further distally than the main bronchus.

E   The tube may be helpful if artificial ventilation is needed.

XVI.12   FTTFF

A   The letters and numbers are correct – but misconnected: *C5–T1.* If you marked this as 'true' it is almost certainly because you disobeyed the only piece of advice that we can give you that really matters and will really make a difference to your score: *read the question.*

D   The three *trunks* form the six divisions at the lateral border of the first rib. The cords are more distal.

E   The median nerve has contributions from the lateral and medial cords; the ulnar nerve is the continuation of the medial cord.

XVI.13   FTTTF

A   This is perhaps a little unfair: there is a muscular sling, but the diaphragm is striated muscle.

C   Under normal circumstances the abdominal pressure acts to close the oesophageal lumen. If pressure is too high, competence is lessened.

E   Abdominal pressures affect ventilation, but airway pressures do not affect the oesophago-gastric junction.

XVI.14   FFFTT

A   The mandibular nerve exits by the foramen ovale. The middle meningeal artery passes through the foramen spinosum.

B   The needle is slipped posteriorly off the lateral pterygoid plate.

C   It is a mixed nerve: motor to the muscles of mastication.

E   The innervation of the skin of the temple is jointly with the zygomatic branch of the ophthalmic division.

XVI.15   FTFTF

Questions about the recurrent laryngeal nerves are asked commonly (see Q XI.16).

A   Bilateral damage causes dysphonia and dyspnoea, but not aphonia.

C   Tetany is caused by low ionised plasma calcium. The *association* between recurrent laryngeal nerve damage and tetany is parathyroid surgery, but that is not *causation.*

E   The cords remain adducted by the cricothyroid muscles, innervated by the superior laryngeal nerve.

XVI.16 FFTTT

Hyperkalaemia causes atrioventricular conduction defects, peaked T waves and *decreased* amplitude of the P waves.

XVI.17 TTFFT

A   *Hypo*tension and *hyper*tension are complications of an acute myocardial infarction.

C,D   Ventriculo-septal defect and ventricular aneurysm are *not common*.

XVI.18 TTTFT

D   The ST segment shows the 'reverse-tick' in patients taking digitalis. The onset of toxicity is not indicated in any specific way in the ECG.

XVI.19 FTTTF

A   Adult panhypopituitarism is *Simmonds'* disease. Sheehan's *syndrome* is hypopituitarism caused by infarction of the pituitary secondary to bleeding in labour. Do you need to know these eponyms? No. But if you didn't, the correct answer is 'don't know'.

E   Glucocorticoids are needed, but not mineralocorticoids.

XVI.20 TTFTT

There is no reason why haemophilia should make syncope likely. Syncope occurs in the other conditions because of:

A   autonomic neuropathy;

B   fixed cardiac output;

D   failure of venous return;

E   peripheral vasodilation and pooling.

XVI.21 TFTTF

B   Intussusception is not a cause of persistent diarrhoea. It may cause obstruction.

D   *Giardia* and amoebiasis infections are common causes of persistent diarrhoea in travellers returned from abroad.

E   Hypokalaemia causes constipation.

XVI.22   FTTTF

 A   Coagulation is a secondary effect.
 D   Platelet contact releases prostaglandin endoperoxidase and thromboxane, both of which alter platelet shape.
 E   Serotonin is not a factor in primary haemostasis.

XVI.23   FTFTT

These are rare syndromes, but matter to anaesthetists.
 A,C   Patients with myasthenic syndrome may be more sensitive than those with myasthenia gravis to depolarising drugs, but there is no difference in response to non-depolarisers.

XVI.24   FTFTF

 A   Coma is *common* only in children.
 C   The level is correct but it is a forced *alkaline* diuresis (did you read the question?): the alkaline urine ionises the salicylate, preventing reabsorption and thus speeding excretion.
 E   This is a difficult MCQ. Aspirin has complex effects on acid-base balance. Acidosis or alkalosis occur, at different times after ingestion. The safe answer, without more detail in the question, might be 'don't know'. But we give the correct answer as 'false', taking 'usual' to mean that any patient who has taken an overdose is expected to be acidotic. That is not so.

XVI.25   TTFFF

 C   Heparin is given first. Warfarin may be started at the same time, but is not first-line treatment.
 D   There is no indication for steroids.
 E   Few of the symptoms and signs in pulmonary embolus are reliable; the X-ray is not an exception.

XVI.26   FTTFF

If ever there was a stock question in all postgraduate medical exams it is this: causes of hilar lymphadenopathy.
 A   Tubercular lymphadenopathy tends to be unilateral.
 D   Diffuse lung lesions, not lymphadenopathy, are diagnostic of pneumoconiosis.
 E   Hilar lymphadenopathy is not a diagnostic feature of SLE.

XVI.27   TTTTF

 E   *Hypo*kalaemia results from persistent vomiting and associated bowel disturbances.

XVI.28   TFTFT

Pain and pallor are the earliest symptoms and signs of acute occlusion; the foot will not take long to become cold. Paralysis takes a little longer to develop as nerve conduction fails.

D   Hydrostatic pressure in the leg will be low: oedema is a sign of *venous* occlusion. Swelling due to compartment syndrome may follow revascularisation.

XVI.29   FFTFF

A   The gallbladder is usually impalpable.

B   Pain usually occurs first (and often suddenly).

D   Early surgery is becoming increasingly popular, but the condition will often resolve spontaneously and allow discharge before elective surgery.

E   Serum liver enzymes soon become abnormal, but liver function remains normal for some time.

XVI.30   FFTFT

A   Most bladder ruptures are caused by trauma. The bladder is more likely to rupture after a direct blow if it is full.

B   A painful desire to pass urine is strangury. Rupture of the bladder is not a cause.

D   Passing any catheter, small or large, will do more damage.

Paper XVII Questions

XVII.1 **If ventilation is impossible after apparently successful intubation, this could be caused by:**
A   kinking of the endotracheal tube in the oropharynx
B   impaction of the endotracheal tube on the carina
C   right endobronchial intubation
D   herniation of the cuff
E   an anaphylactoid drug response.

XVII.2 **Immediate treatment of a postoperative thyrotoxic crisis includes:**
A   sedation with chlorpromazine
B   active rewarming
C   intravenous steroids
D   propranolol
E   carbimazole.

XVII.3 **In blind-nasal intubation:**
A   carbon dioxide can be added to the inspired gas mixture to facilitate intubation
B   halothane should not be used for anaesthesia as it can cause cardiac arrhythmias
C   the tube may pass into the oesophagus if the neck is excessively flexed
D   mucosal laceration over the arch of the atlas is a common cause of bleeding
E   thiopentone is contraindicated as an induction agent.

XVII.4 **Awareness during anaesthesia:**
A   is a problem only in unpremedicated patients
B   is recognised by constriction of the pupil
C   is associated with tachycardia and production of tears
D   is prevented in most patients by 0.5% isoflurane in 60% nitrous oxide
E   is associated with an altered sensation of pain.

XVII.5 **An asymptomatic patient presenting for elective hysterectomy has a haemoglobin concentration of 9 g/dl. You should:**

A delay surgery and investigate the anaemia
B transfuse the patient with packed cells preoperatively
C proceed with anaesthesia and surgery, but transfuse the patient with blood intraoperatively if required
D arrange for clotting factors and platelets to be available in case the patient bleeds postoperatively
E use higher inspired oxygen concentrations than usual during anaesthesia.

XVII.6 **Late complications of nasotracheal intubation include:**

A deafness
B maxillary abscess
C sloughing of the pharyngeal mucosal
D necrosis of alar cartilage
E transient cranial mononeuropathy of the left recurrent laryngeal nerve.

XVII.7 **Appropriate treatment of air embolism occurring during posterior fossa surgery includes:**

A jugular compression
B increasing the mean intrathoracic pressure
C aspiration via a central venous catheter
D a mannitol infusion
E turning the patient on to the left side head down.

XVII.8 **A 35-year-old primigravida is induced at 37 weeks because of pre-eclampsia. She is complaining of tingling in her fingers but is otherwise asymptomatic. The following would be reasons for avoiding epidural analgesia:**

A a diastolic blood pressure above 120 mmHg
B persistent fetal tachycardia
C signs of disordered blood clotting
D heavy proteinuria
E refusal by the patient.

XVII.9 **A healthy 6-week-old baby presents with pyloric stenosis, and requires general anaesthesia for Ramstedt's operation. A suitable anaesthetic technique could include:**

A intravenous induction with thiopentone
B intubation under neuromuscular blockade with atracurium
C 0.3 mg intramuscular atropine as premedication
D intravenous fluid therapy with sodium chloride
E use of a size 1 laryngeal mask airway.

XVII.10   Nitrous oxide:
A   does not combine with haemoglobin
B   produces increased tension in a pneumothorax
C   induces bone marrow aplasia
D   is partially metabolised by intestinal bacteria
E   causes diffusion hypoxia at the termination of anaesthesia.

XVII.11   In the detection of abnormal serum cholinesterase:
A   dibucaine inhibits serum cholinesterase
B   97% of the population possess the normal enzyme
C   the dibucaine number is more than 80 in patients homozygous for the abnormal enzyme
D   the dibucaine number is about 60 in patients who are heterozygous for the abnormal enzyme
E   fluoride is used as an alternative enzyme inhibitor.

XVII.12   After pneumonectomy:
A   a single chest drain is commonly used
B   chest drainage must be allowed to bubble freely
C   a Maxwell box may be used to centralise the mediastinum
D   tension pneumothorax is a common cause of hypotension
E   there is often surgical emphysema.

XVII.13   The cephalic vein:
A   is one of the major deep veins of the upper limb
B   communicates with the basilic vein via the median cubital vein
C   at the elbow lies between brachioradialis and biceps
D   in the upper arm lies in the delto-pectoral groove
E   drains directly into the axillary vein.

XVII.14   The dura mater:
A   is a double membrane extending from within the cranium to the filum terminale
B   is attached above to the edges of the foramen magnum
C   is attached posteriorly by the posterior longitudinal ligament
D   encloses the dural sac down to the level of approximately the second sacral segment
E   at spinal level is lined by the arachnoid mater.

XVII.15   The glossopharyngeal nerve:

A   supplies all pharyngeal sensation except for the tonsil
B   supplies sensation to the posterior third of the tongue
C   passes through the jugular foramen
D   supplies fibres to the otic ganglion
E   carries afferent information from the carotid sinus.

XVII.16   Cervical plexus block:

A   is effective with about 4 ml of 1.5% lignocaine at the transverse processes of C3–5
B   if performed bilaterally, and combined with a light general anaesthetic, gives a good, bloodless field for thyroidectomy
C   is likely to cause a Horner's syndrome
D   is best performed avoiding solutions containing adrenaline
E   may result in dural puncture as a recognised complication.

XVII.17   In the electrocardiogram:

A   the QT interval varies with the plasma calcium
B   a prolonged QT interval occurs in hypokalaemia
C   hypokalaemia is accompanied by ST depression
D   biphasic P waves occur with extreme hyperkalaemia
E   the PR interval is short in Wolff–Parkinson–White syndrome.

XVII.18   Causes of atrial fibrillation include:

A   sarcoidosis
B   rheumatic heart disease
C   cardiomyopathy
D   hypertension
E   atropine administration.

XVII.19   In malignant hypertension, there is an increased likelihood of:

A   cerebral haemorrhage
B   renal failure
C   congestive cardiac failure
D   left ventricular failure
E   pulmonary hypertension.

XVII.20 **When glucocorticoid plasma concentrations are increased there is:**
  A   dehydration
  B   hypertension
  C   muscle weakness
  D   potassium depletion
  E   osteoporosis.

XVII.21 **Hypothermia:**
  A   may develop during chlorpromazine therapy
  B   occurs in acute pancreatitis
  C   causes unconsciousness when core temperature drops to 33°C
  D   causes a 'J' wave in the electrocardiogram
  E   is likely to occur intraoperatively at the extremes of age.

XVII.22 **Causes of intestinal malabsorption include:**
  A   coeliac disease
  B   hyperparathyroidism
  C   diabetes mellitus
  D   carcinoid syndrome
  E   tropical sprue.

XVII.23 **Dystrophia myotonica:**
  A   is a primary disorder of the myoneural junction
  B   is associated with cataract formation
  C   is associated with gonadal atrophy
  D   only occurs in males
  E   is associated with limb weakness.

XVII.24 **The following statements about oral hypoglycaemic drugs are true:**
  A   chlorpropamide has a half-life of 36 hours
  B   metformin increases lactic acid production
  C   dangerous hypoglycaemia does not occur
  D   the duration of action of glibenclamide is less than 6 hours
  E   sulphonylurea and biguanide drugs should not be given concurrently.

XVII.25 **In polycystic disease of the kidney:**
  A   inheritance is an autosomal dominant
  B   presentation is usually in middle adult life
  C   pyelonephritis is a common complication
  D   hypertension is a common complication
  E   life expectancy is little reduced provided the patients follow a renal diet.

XVII.26   **Associations of primary carcinoma of the lung include:**
A   inappropriate secretion of antidiuretic hormone
B   hyperglycaemia
C   Horner's syndrome
D   hypertrophic pulmonary osteoarthropathy
E   carcinoid syndrome.

XVII.27   **A 58-year-old man is brought into casualty with 35% burns, having poured methylated spirit on to a lighted barbecue. He is conscious, in pain and distressed:**
A   opioids should be avoided
B   an intravenous infusion of 5% dextrose should be started immediately
C   if he needs an anaesthetic for immediate escharotomy he must not be given suxamethonium
D   an oximeter will give an accurate indication of arterial saturation
E   serial haematocrit measurement is a good aid to fluid replacement.

XVII.28   **The following are true of traumatic rupture of the spleen:**
A   patients whose spleens are removed after traumatic rupture are not at risk of subsequent pneumococcal pneumonias
B   it is more likely if the patient has malaria
C   the abdomen is soft if no other viscera is injured
D   rupture can be delayed more than 14 days
E   radiological signs include obliteration of the psoas shadow.

XVII.29   **The following are true of rupture of the oesophagus:**
A   the patient is usually surprisingly well
B   prognosis is better in spontaneous rupture than rupture after instrumentation
C   surgical emphysema is a common sign
D   the need for surgical repair is extremely urgent
E   a barium swallow may be helpful if there is doubt in diagnosis.

XVII.30   **Following the prolapse of an intervertebral disc:**
A   if at L4–5 there will be weakness of ankle dorsiflexion
B   if at L4–5 the ankle jerk will be preserved
C   if at L5–S1 there will be pain in the calf
D   bladder symptoms are an indication for urgent surgery
E   a steroid epidural offers the best chance of cure.

Paper XVII Answers

XVII.1 TFFTT
- **B** The angle of the carina is too sharp to obstruct the whole of the lumen of the tube.
- **C** The right lung should ventilate easily.
- **E** Not all anaphylactic responses cause bronchospasm; if it happens, treat with adrenaline rapidly.

XVII.2 TFTTT

Note the word 'immediate'.
- **A,** Chlorpromazine, dexamethasone, propranolol and
- **C–E** carbimazole are all recommended as part of the early treatment in the *Oxford Handbook of Clinical Medicine*. Lugol's iodine and fluids can also be given.
- **B** The patient will need to be *cooled* by tepid sponging.

XVII.3 TFTFF

The fibreoptic laryngoscope means that fewer trainees see this technique nowadays, but it has its advocates.
- **A** The standard method was to add 1–2 *litres* per minute to the fresh gas flow: historically this is why such high flows of carbon dioxide are available.
- **B** Halothane does cause ventricular ectopic beats, especially if there is hypercapnia, but it has been used successfully during numerous blind nasal intubations.
- **D** This laceration can occur – but it is not a *common* cause of bleeding. The commonest cause is minor trauma in the nasal passages.
- **E** Not so, provided intubation is not attempted on thiopentone alone.

XVII.4 FFTTF
- **A** Premedication reduces but does not prevent the possibility of awareness. Drugs with powerful amnesic properties, such as lorazepam, may prevent recall.
- **B** Pupils are more likely to dilate.
- **C** Tachycardia and tears are not invariable.
- **D** Usually this combination prevents awareness, but a few patients, notably alcoholics and drug addicts, may remain aware.
- **E** Patients can certainly be aware but not in pain, despite surgery continuing. Whether or not this is truly altered sensation of pain does not affect the answer: patients can be aware and in pain.

XVII.5   FFTFF

A,B   When the first edition of this book was written the answer to these questions would have been 'true'; times and advice change and the recommended lower limit for haemoglobin concentrations in asymptomatic chronic anaemia is now 8 g/dl.

D   This patient is not at increased risk of clotting disorders.

E   The anaemia is not severe enough that increased inspired oxygen will make any important difference to oxygen carriage.

XVII.6   TTTTT

E   Sounds wonderful and is true, though rather rare!

XVII.7   TTTFT

D   Mannitol may be used if cerebral swelling occurs as a result of air embolism, but it is not a treatment for the condition.

E   Turning the patient into this position is standard advice. It is usually impossible halfway through an operation.

XVII.8   FFTFT

Epidural analgesia is recommended in pre-eclampsia, and early in labour rather than late.

A   Because pre-eclampsia is a disease of the small vessels, the blood pressure may not decrease if the condition is severe. That is not a reason for avoiding an epidural.

B,D   These are both irrelevant to an epidural.

E   The patient must always be asked. You can try to persuade but, although current opinion is that epidural analgesia is of benefit in pre-eclampsia, this does not allow over-riding of the mother's wishes (see Q XV.8).

XVII.9   TTFTF

A   A 6-week-old baby will probably be a bit vigorous for an awake intubation. There is a school of thought that condemns awake intubation (see Q I.9).

B   Some anaesthetists always use suxamethonium when there is pyloric stenosis; others think that atracurium works quickly enough in this age group.

C   A dose of 0.3 mg atropine is too much: the usual dose is 0.015 mg/kg (see Q I.9).

D   Pyloric stenosis is not an emergency: fluid resuscitation comes first.

E   A laryngeal mask airway does not protect against regurgitation and is unsuitable in cases of intestinal obstruction.

XVII.10   TTTTT

These are all true, though the effect on bone marrow does not matter unless exposure lasts for many hours.

XVII.11   TTFTT

C,D   It is easy to get the association of degree of inhibition and abnormality of enzyme the wrong way round. Homozygous patients possess only abnormal enzyme. This is dibucaine *resistant*, so that inhibition, at 16–20%, is *less* than normal, which is 80%.

XVII.12   TFTFF

B   The chest drain is clamped to prevent mediastinal movement.

C   You cannot know everything. This is small print stuff. A Maxwell box (an external device used to regulate the volume of air in the chest and keep the mediastinum central) is a long way down the list of things needed to be known to gain the FRCA.

D   Tension pneumothorax is unlikely, provided the drain is clamped.

E   Surgical emphysema is rare.

XVII.13   FTTTT

A   The cephalic vein is superficial. Most of the venous drainage of the arm is through superficial veins.

D   The delto-pectoral groove is a site for percutaneous puncture and direct cut-down.

XVII.14   FTFTT

A   The dura mater is double only inside the cranium, the two layers enclosing the cerebral sinuses.

C   It is attached *anteriorly* to the posterior longitudinal ligament.

XVII.15   FTTTT

A   The glossopharyngeal nerve innervates the tonsil as well.

D   Parasympathetic fibres go to the otic ganglion via the lesser superficial petrosal nerve.

XVII.16   TFTTT

The neck is tiger country so: avoid adrenaline (**D**); aspirate carefully (**D,E**); and bilateral block (**B**) should not be undertaken lightly (it can result in bilateral phrenic paralysis).

XVII.17   TTTTT

XVII.18   TTTTF

A   Small print, but atrial fibrillation and sarcoidosis is a recognised association.

E   Atropine does not cause atrial fibrillation. Slow atrial fibrillation may even revert to sinus rhythm when atropine is given (though this is a casual observation, not a suggested treatment for fibrillation).

XVII.19   TTFTF

C,E   In malignant hypertension, the problem is left-sided.

XVII.20   FTTTT

Increased glucocorticoids cause Cushing's syndrome, which may be endogenous or iatrogenic.

A   There is usually fluid retention and oedema.

XVII.21   TFFTT

A   Hypothermia can develop because of vasodilation.

B   Shock yes: but in acute pancreatitis hypothermia is not a specific sign.

C   Patients may be weak and confused at 33°C; consciousness is lost at about 31°C.

D   A 'J' wave may follow the QRS complex.

XVII.22   TFTTT

B,C   These are small print, though diabetes is an important disease. Hyperparathyroidism causes intestinal malabsorption.

A,D,   These three are easier questions – though carcinoid is
E   rare (but often asked about in anaesthesia exams) and tropical sprue is not a common disease in Europe.

XVII.23   FTTTT

A   Dystrophia myotonica is a disorder of the muscle fibres themselves, not the myoneural junction.

XVII.24   TTFFF

C   Dangerous hypoglycaemia can occur. It may be difficult to diagnose in the elderly.

D   The duration of action of glibenclamide is 12–16 hours.

E   Combination therapy is recommended in certain circumstances for patients with stable non-ketotic non-insulin-dependent diabetes.

XVII.25   TTTTF

B   There is a rarer infantile form of polycystic disease.

E   Life expectancy is reduced in polycystic disease of the kidneys.

XVII.26   TFTTT

    B   Hypoglycaemia is associated with lung cancer.

    C   Carcinomas at the apex of the lung, Pancoast tumours, can affect the brachial plexus and recurrent laryngeal nerve.

    D   A complicated name for 'clubbing' of nails.

XVII.27   FFFFT

    A   Opioids can be given with care.

    B   Plasma or saline should be given: certainly not dextrose.

    C   Suxamethonium can be used immediately after the incident. Classically, suxamethonium causes abrupt hyperkalaemia 3–5 weeks later.

    D   Burned patients may have clinically important amounts of carboxyhaemoglobin, which is 'seen' by the oximeter as oxygenated blood.

XVII.28   FTFTT

    A   All patients who have had a splenectomy should take precautions against pneumococcal pneumonia.

    C   Over half the patients show rigidity.

    D   Late delayed rupture is not common, but certainly occurs.

    E   The psoas shadow disappears because of overlying blood.

XVII.29   FFTTF

    A,B A patient whose oesophagus has ruptured is usually in great distress, especially after spontaneous rupture. This usually follows vomiting, and gastric contents in the mediastinum will make the patient very ill.

    E   Lipiodol yes, barium no: it is an irritant to the mediastinal tissues.

XVII.30   TTTTF

When there are segmental symptoms and imaging evidence of a disc protrusion, surgery is the best chance of cure.

    E   Steroid epidurals can provide symptomatic relief, whether this is a cure is debatable.

Paper XVIII Questions

XVIII.1 Appropriate treatment for hypotension following induction with propofol includes:
A glycopyrronium
B 1 litre Hartmann's solution
C phentolamine
D ephedrine
E ergometrine.

XVIII.2 In an adult who is bleeding briskly 48 h after elective adeno-tonsillectomy:
A shock is unlikely to be severe
B surgery should be delayed for 4 hours after the patient last ate food
C the patient's serum should be grouped and saved before induction of anaesthesia
D gaseous induction is mandatory
E cricoid pressure is of no benefit because the bleeding is from above the glottis.

XVIII.3 In men over 50 years of age, the statistical probability of a myocardial infarction occurring in the postoperative period is:
A decreased if a high inspired oxygen concentration is used during anaesthesia
B increased if there is a history of myocardial infarction within the past 6 months
C increased by prolongation of surgery
D increased with perioperative evidence of ST segment depression
E increased with preoperative history of angina.

XVIII.4   Perioperative management of a jaundiced patient about to undergo diagnostic laparotomy should include:

A   a clotting screen
B   a mannitol infusion
C   prophylactic antibiotics
D   thromboembolic prophylaxis with subcutaneous heparin
E   vasopressin therapy to reduce risk of bleeding from varices.

XVIII.5   Suitable sedative techniques for use in intensive care include:

A   thiopentone infusion
B   midazolam infusion
C   morphine infusion
D   etomidate infusion
E   propofol infusion.

XVIII.6   Elective hypotension in neurosurgery:

A   is satisfactorily achieved with halothane and mechanical ventilation
B   is contraindicated in surgery for intracranial aneurysm
C   affects autoregulation of the cerebral circulation
D   is associated with a reduction in cerebral oxygenation
E   increases the risk of air embolism.

XVIII.7   Appropriate prophylaxis against the acid-aspiration syndrome includes:

A   mist. magnesium trisilicate
B   ondansetron
C   hydrocortisone
D   intravenous H_2-antagonist
E   sodium citrate.

XVIII.8   Appropriate treatment in a patient thought to have suffered an amniotic fluid embolus includes:

A   blood transfusion
B   heparin
C   ephedrine
D   steroids
E   salbutamol.

XVIII.9   The following are true of thiopentone:

A   the drug is highly acidic when mixed with water
B   hypotension due to vasodilation is common
C   extravascular injection can cause cutaneous sloughing
D   its use can precipitate an attack of porphyria
E   it is the agent of choice in asthmatics.

XVIII.10 **Features of anaesthesia with desflurane include:**
A rapid induction of anaesthesia
B potentiation of muscle relaxants
C reduction in intracranial pressure
D analgesia that lasts into the postoperative period
E moderate hypotension.

XVIII.11 **Bronchospasm complicating anaesthesia can occur with the administration of:**
A suxamethonium
B etomidate
C dextrans
D metoclopramide given rapidly intravenously
E whole blood.

XVIII.12 **The following are true of the muscles of the pharynx:**
A the superior constrictor is stylopharyngeus
B cricopharyngeus is the inferior part of the lower constrictor and is composed of transverse fibres
C cricopharyngeus functions as a sphincter
D pharyngeal pouches tend to occur anteriorly through the lower constrictor
E the constrictor muscles are supplied by nerve fibres from the vagus and glossopharyngeal nerves.

XVIII.13 **When the brachial plexus is anaesthetised by the supraclavicular route:**
A the aim is to deposit local anaesthetic solution around the trunks as they emerge from beneath the first rib
B a total of 15 ml 2% lignocaine with adrenaline should be sufficient
C a nerve stimulator risks pleural burns
D an upper arm tourniquet will not cause pain
E the palmar skin occasionally is not fully anaesthetised.

XVIII.14 **The following are true of nerves supplying extraocular muscles:**
A an oculomotor palsy causes loss of the accommodation reflex
B an oculomotor palsy causes enophthalmos and ptosis
C a trochlear palsy causes diplopia when looking down and out
D a VIth nerve palsy causes a divergent squint
E the VIth nerve has an extremely thin connective tissue sheath.

XVIII.15   The lateral popliteal (common peroneal) nerve:

    A subserves sensation on the dorsum of the foot via the musculocutaneous (superficial peroneal) nerve
    B subserves sensation over the whole of the dorsum of the foot
    C is a sensory nerve
    D supplies the skin over a variable area of the lateral lower leg
    E ends as the anterior tibial and medial calcaneal nerves.

XVIII.16   Hypokalaemia is a recognised feature of:

    A diarrhoea
    B excess mineralocorticoid secretion
    C triamterene therapy
    D metabolic alkalosis
    E uretero-colic anastomosis.

XVIII.17   Common causes of pericarditis include:

    A viral infection
    B acute myocardial infarction
    C pulmonary embolism
    D tuberculosis
    E uraemia.

XVIII.18   The maintenance dose of digoxin should be reduced:

    A in thyrotoxicosis
    B after myocardial infarction
    C if there is impaired renal function
    D for cardiopulmonary bypass
    E in the elderly.

XVIII.19   A diastolic cardiac murmur occurs in:

    A mitral incompetence
    B ventricular septal defect
    C aortic regurgitation
    D atrio-septal defect
    E patent ductus arteriosus.

XVIII.20   Likely problems in a patient suffering from hypothyroidism include:

    A prolonged effect of opioids
    B hypoglycaemia
    C hypothermia
    D positive Trousseau's sign
    E prolonged response to non-depolarising neuromuscular blocking drugs.

XVIII.21 **The following are true of Crohn's disease:**
A it affects predominantly females
B it affects only the terminal ileum
C it is more likely than ulcerative colitis to lead to fistulae
D it is associated with uveitis
E it commonly presents with bloody diarrhoea.

XVIII.22 **The following occur in haemophilia:**
A haemarthrosis
B prolonged bleeding time
C prolonged partial thromboplastin time
D impaired clot retraction
E a haemorrhagic skin rash.

XVIII.23 **In patients with myasthenia gravis:**
A there is insensitivity to non-depolarising muscle relaxants
B 15% will have a thymoma
C ophthalmoplegia may be the only symptom
D blood gases are a good guide to ventilatory function
E pyridostigmine overdose does not cause a depolarisation block.

XVIII.24 **Common findings in patients with acute renal failure include:**
A metabolic acidosis
B hyperkalaemia
C anaemia
D decreased circulating fluid volume
E cerebral oedema.

XVIII.25 **Reduced total lung compliance is commonly associated with:**
A left ventricular failure
B emphysema
C kyphoscoliosis
D pulmonary fibrosis
E asthma.

XVIII.26   A 35-year-old asthmatic woman, who usually uses salbutamol and beclomethasone inhalers, is brought into casualty acutely dyspnoeic.

A   additional intravenous steroids are contraindicated because they can produce adrenal suppression

B   if her $PaCO_2$ is 4 kPa (30 mmHg) it is probably safe not to start IPPV immediately

C   she should not be given more than 35% oxygen by mask

D   she should lie down to make her breathing easier

E   she will have a prolonged inspiratory time.

XVIII.27   Indications for splenectomy include:

A   schistosomiasis

B   idiopathic thrombocytopenic purpura

C   spontaneous rupture due to infectious mononucleosis

D   Hodgkin's disease

E   hereditary spherocytosis.

XVIII.28   Features of chronic pyloric obstruction include:

A   tetany

B   visible peristalsis

C   postural hypotension

D   hypokalaemia

E   epigastric succussion splash.

XVIII.29 **Likely complications of laparoscopy include:**
  A   hypotension
  B   bradycardia
  C   shoulder pain
  D   gas embolism
  E   deep venous thrombosis.

XVIII.30 **The absorption of large quantities of glycine during prolonged transurethral prostatic resection can produce:**
  A   hyponatraemia
  B   haemolysis
  C   haemodilution
  D   hyperkalaemia
  E   hypoglycaemia.

Paper XVIII Answers

XVIII.1 TTFTF

A A bradycardia is common and may require treatment with a vagolytic drug.

B The hypotension is usually due to a decreased systemic vascular resistance, which fluid loading can help to counter.

C Phentolamine is an alpha blocker, which will induce vasodilation.

D Ephedrine will cause peripheral vasoconstriction and an increase in heart rate: the desired effects.

E Ergometrine is used as an oxytocic and not for its vasoconstricting action.

XVIII.2 FFFFF

Question XII.2 is also about this common exam topic.

A Patients of all ages can still bleed to death after tonsillectomy.

B This is a useless and possibly hazardous precaution because the patient will continue to swallow blood.

C In a patient with 'brisk haemorrhage', blood should be cross-matched.

D Gaseous induction is often recommended in children, but in all age groups can be difficult if bleeding is brisk. Many experienced anaesthetists prefer an intravenous induction.

E A lot of blood will have been swallowed and cricoid pressure may prevent this being regurgitated.

XVIII.3 FTFTT

A High inspired oxygen concentrations do not affect the probability of infarction unless necessary to maintain adequate oxygenation, which would be in seriously ill patients only.

B Recent myocardial infarction increases the risk of anaesthesia. The risk returns to normal in a patient who has been asymptomatic for 3 years.

C Prolonged surgery may cause more pulmonary problems, but not myocardial infarction.

XVIII.4 TTTFF

B   Mannitol is given to lessen the likelihood of hepato-renal syndrome.

D   The safe answer is 'false', although not all jaundiced patients have disturbed clotting, and heparin may be indicated.

E   Vasopressin is not prophylaxis for varices (and nor do all jaundiced patients have varices, a complication of raised portal vein pressure not of jaundice).

XVIII.5 TTTFT

A–C,   All these drugs are used in various situations. Propofol

E   infusions should not be used in young children.

D   Etomidate is not used because of the associated adrenocortical suppression.

XVIII.6 FFTTF

A   This is not satisfactory because the concentration of halothane needed would increase cerebral blood flow.

D   Not when hypotension is caused by elective vasodilation.

E   Arterial hypotension does not affect venous pressure.

XVIII.7 FFFTT

A   Another case of times changing: the answer in the first edition was 'true', but because it is a particulate antacid mist. mag. trisil. is no longer recommended .

B   Ondansetron is an antiemetic but it does not affect acidity or regurgitation.

C   Hydrocortisone is not a prophylactic measure.

D H_2-antagonists do not have an immediate effect. They are given with a suitable antacid.

XVIII.8 TTTTT

B   A coagulopathy is likely and heparin can be useful. It is a good idea to involve the haematologists because clotting disorders can be complex and they tend to change character rapidly.

XVIII.9 FTTTF

A   Thiopentone is an acid, but is strongly alkaline when made up. It should not be mixed with other anaesthetic drugs.

E   Thiopentone is said to be contraindicated because of laryngeal sensitisation and bronchospasm.

XVIII.10   TTFFT

C   Intracranial pressure is increased. Desflurane should not be used in neurosurgical patients.
D   Desflurane is minimally metabolised and has no persistent analgesic effects.

XVIII.11   TFTFT

A   Neuromuscular blocking agents are the anaesthetic drugs most likely to cause bronchospasm, and suxamethonium certainly can.
B,D   You could say that any drug 'can' cause bronchospasm, but clinical experience shows that etomidate and metoclopramide are not important causes.
C,E   Dextran solutions and blood products can cause allergic-type reactions.

XVIII.12   TTTFF

B,C   The transverse fibres of cricopharyngeus form a sphincter.
D   Pharyngeal pouches tend to occur posterolaterally between the functionally different upper and lower fibres.
E   Innervation is from the vagal and *accessory* nerves.

XVIII.13   FFFFT

A   The trunks *cross* the first rib.
B   This volume is too little: 30–40 ml 1–2% lignocaine with adrenaline.
C   Using a stimulator improves the success rate. The comment about pleural burns is a red herring.
D   Analgesia of the inner aspect of the upper arm is not guaranteed.
E   The median nerve (middle trunk, C7) sometimes escapes.

XVIII.14   TFTTF

A   The pupillary constrictor is paralysed.
B   Ptosis only, enophthalmos and ptosis occur in a Horner's (SNS paralysis).
E   The VIth nerve is vulnerable because of its long course.

XVIII.15   TTFTF

B,E   The anterior tibial *is* a branch of the lateral popliteal. The medial calcaneal is a cutaneous branch of the *posterior* tibial and supplies the heel.

C   The lateral popliteal is a mixed nerve: it contains sensory and motor fibres. When a nerve is described as a sensory nerve, it means that it contains only sensory fibres.

XVIII.16   TTFTT

C   Triamterene is an aldosterone antagonist, so potassium is conserved at the expense of sodium.

E   Urine in the colon decreases transit time and therefore increases potassium excretion.

XVIII.17   TTFFT

C,D   The question includes the word 'commonly' and should be assumed to apply to practice in the Western world unless stated otherwise. Tuberculosis may re-emerge as a common cause.

XVIII.18   FFTTT

A   In thyrotoxicosis, treat the thyroid problem.

B   After an infarction, it may be deleterious to reduce the dose.

D   Digoxin is usually stopped before cardiac surgery because defibrillation of a digitalised heart is less effective.

XVIII.19   FTTFF

A   Mitral incompetence causes a systolic murmur; mitral stenosis a diastolic murmur.

E   A ductus causes a continuous machinery murmur, not a diastolic murmur.

XVIII.20   TTTFT

D   Trousseau's sign, which occurs in hypo*parathyroidism*, is the '*main d'accoucheur*' hand position produced by inflating a tourniquet cuff above arterial pressure in a patient with hypocalcaemic tetany.

XVIII.21   FFTTF

    A   Men and women are equally affected by Crohn's disease.

    B   Although commonest in the terminal ileum, it can affect any part of the gastrointestinal tract from mouth to anus.

    D   Uveitis and iritis are both associations.

    E   Diarrhoea is common, but it is uncommon for the motions to contain frank blood, which is a feature of ulcerative colitis.

XVIII.22   TTFFF

    C   Partial thromboplastin time tests the intrinsic pathway and the prothrombin-dependent factors.

    D   Clot retraction is a platelet-dependent effect.

    E   Skin rashes are not a feature of haemophilia.

XVIII.23   TTTFF

    A   They are very sensitive to the effects of these drugs and reduced dosage is needed.

    C   In some patients with ophthalmoplegia the disease never progresses.

    D   Change in blood gases are a late result of ventilatory failure in myasthenia.

    E   Pyridostigmine is longer-acting than neostigmine. Both can cause depolarisation block in relative excess.

XVIII.24   TTTFT

    D   Circulating fluid volume will be normal or increased in acute renal failure.

XVIII.25   TFTTF

Total lung compliance is measured when there is no airflow through the airways.

    B   Compliance increases in emphysema.

    E   Compliance is not reduced in asthma. Airway resistance is much increased.

XVIII.26   FTFFF

The British Thoracic Society has produced guidelines on the management of asthma.

A   Steroids are the mainstay of treatment and doses will have to be increased during the acute phase of the attack.

B   The $PaCO_2$ is usually low in acute asthma. A *normal* $PaCO_2$ is a sign that IPPV may be needed.

C   She should be given humidified oxygen in high concentration.

D   Breathing is likely to be easier sitting up.

E   Expiratory time is prolonged.

XVIII.27   FTTTT

Splenectomy is not the benign operation it was thought to be. Patients without a spleen are at high risk of certain infections (see Q. XVII.28).

A   Splenomegaly is a complication of schistosomiasis, but is not treated operatively.

B   Removing the spleen in idiopathic thrombocytopenic purpura helps to preserve the platelets.

D   Splenectomy is part of a staging laparotomy in lymphomas, but probably does not affect outcome. It is much less popular than 10 years ago because of improvements in intra-abdominal imaging.

XVIII.28   TFFTT

Effective treatment of peptic ulcers has made this condition much less common than 20 years ago.

A   The metabolic alkalosis decreases the plasma ionised calcium.

B   Visible peristalsis is a feature of acute lower bowel obstruction.

C   There is no association between postural hypotension and chronic pyloric obstruction.

E   Succussion splash is a classical surgical sign. There are many similar signs in medicine, and they are being gradually forgotten as investigational techniques become more sophisticated and more commonly available.

XVIII.29   TTTFF

Note the inclusion of the word 'likely'.
D,E   Both have been reported, but are they *likely* in your
experience?

XVIII.30   TFTFT

A,C,   All are dilutional, caused by absorption of isotonic
E   fluid (usually glycine) that contains no electrolyte.
B   Haemolysis will not occur with isotonic fluid.
D   Dilution would produce hypokalaemia.

Paper XIX Questions

XIX.1 **In the following conditions, a temporary pacemaker should be inserted preoperatively:**
  A complete heart block
  B atrial flutter with 2:1 block
  C right bundle branch block with left axis deviation
  D Stokes–Adams attacks
  E multiple ventricular extrasystoles.

XIX.2 **The following are suitable techniques for hypotensive anaesthesia for major head and neck surgery:**
  A intravenous increments of phentolamine
  B labetalol and isoflurane
  C a bolus injection of esmolol
  D an intradural injection of 3.5 ml of 0.5% heavy bupivacaine
  E an infusion of sodium nitroprusside.

XIX.3 **There are occasions when nitrous oxide anaesthesia is contraindicated. These include some patients:**
  A with air embolism
  B with bowel distension caused by intestinal obstruction
  C with pneumothorax
  D undergoing middle ear surgery
  E with pernicious anaemia.

XIX.4   **4 hours after general anaesthesia for elective laparotomy and hemicolectomy, a patient is breathless and distressed with a mild tachycardia and a blood pressure of 170/100 mmHg. Blood gases show PaO_2 9 kPa (70 mmHg), $PaCO_2$ 9 kPa (70 mmHg) and bicarbonate 28 mmol/l. Likely diagnoses include:**
    A   pulmonary segmental collapse
    B   blood loss
    C   metabolic acidosis
    D   over-transfusion
    E   hypoventilation.

XIX.5   **Patients at greater than normal risk of developing Gram-negative septicaemia include those suffering from:**
    A   diabetes mellitus
    B   cirrhosis
    C   leukaemia
    D   polycythaemia
    E   uraemia.

XIX.6   **Common approaches to local anaesthesia of the brachial plexus include:**
    A   axillary
    B   interscalene
    C   infraclavicular
    D   subclavian
    E   supraclavicular.

XIX.7   **Epidural anaesthesia in labour:**
    A   is contraindicated in patients with sickle-cell disease
    B   masks placental abruption
    C   increases placental blood flow
    D   masks uterine rupture
    E   is contraindicated in patients with peripheral neuropathy.

XIX.8   **Suitable techniques to counter the fall in blood pressure at the onset of spinal anaesthesia for caesarean section include:**
    A   preloading with crystalloid
    B   Trendelenburg position
    C   slow injection using a spinal catheter
    D   subcutaneous adrenaline
    E   intravenous ephedrine.

XIX.9 **Suitable methods to help in the relief of postoperative pain after elective gastrectomy include:**
A cryoanalgesia
B intercostal nerve blockade
C epidural chlorocresol
D patient-controlled analgesia with opioid
E sustained-release oral morphine.

XIX.10 **Etomidate is:**
A contraindicated in atopic patients
B rapidly metabolised in the liver
C diabetogenic
D suitable for use in patients with acute intermittent porphyria
E suitable for use in patients with increased intracranial pressure.

XIX.11 **Nitric oxide:**
A is an environmental pollutant with a long half-life
B is an intracellular second messenger
C stimulates platelet aggregation
D is toxic by conversion to nitrogen dioxide
E is a specific vasodilator of the pulmonary circulation.

XIX.12 **A 3-year-old child presents in the accident department, thought to have inhaled a peanut 2 hours previously. A reasonable scheme of anaesthetic management for bronchoscopy and removal of the foreign body includes:**
A premedication with atropine
B gaseous induction with halothane
C the avoidance of nitrous oxide
D use of a ventilating bronchoscope and muscle relaxants
E bronchopulmonary lavage.

XIX.13 **The brachial artery:**
A is readily palpable throughout its length
B is crossed by the bicipital aponeurosis
C is crossed by the median cubital vein
D is crossed from lateral to medial by the median nerve
E divides at the wrist into the ulnar and radial arteries.

XIX.14 Nerves at risk of damage by positioning of patients for surgery include:

  A   median
  B   saphenous
  C   facial
  D   trigeminal
  E   lateral popliteal.

XIX.15 Damage to the sciatic nerve by a misplaced intramuscular injection into the buttock:

  A   can be avoided by using short-bevelled needles
  B   can be avoided if the injection is given anterior to a line joining the posterior superior iliac spine to the greater trochanter
  C   causes anaesthesia over the ischial tuberosity
  D   causes weakness or paralysis of all muscles below the knee
  E   spares the sole of the foot.

XIX.16 Hypernatraemia occurs:

  A   after severe burns
  B   after intravenous feeding with 50% dextrose
  C   in hyperaldosteronism
  D   in renal failure
  E   in cystic fibrosis.

XIX.17 Likely causes of cardiomegaly observed on an anterior–posterior (A–P) chest radiograph include:

  A   congestive cardiac failure
  B   pleural effusion
  C   mitral stenosis
  D   complete heart block
  E   the normal variation in heart size.

XIX.18 A midsystolic ejection murmur is heard in:

  A   aortic stenosis
  B   systemic hypertension
  C   coarctation of the aorta
  D   atrio-septal defect
  E   mitral regurgitation.

XIX.19 **There is a visible 'a' wave in the jugular venous pulse in:**
A   atrial fibrillation
B   first-degree heart block
C   ventricular tachycardia
D   atrial flutter
E   pulmonary embolus.

XIX.20 **A patient presents for elective thyroidectomy. The following are evidence that the patient is clinically hyperthyroid:**
A   the patient is febrile
B   the heart rate is greater than 100 beats/min
C   the patient suffers from stridor
D   signs of right heart failure are present
E   Chvostek's sign is positive.

XIX.21 **Indications for urgent surgical treatment of ulcerative colitis include:**
A   anaemia
B   acute toxic dilation
C   development of pyoderma gangrenosa
D   to avoid the use of steroids
E   severe dehydration caused by intractable diarrhoea.

XIX.22 **The following statements are true of jaundice:**
A   urinary bilirubin is increased in obstructive jaundice
B   urinary urobilinogen is decreased in hepatocellular jaundice
C   there is normal urinary urobilinogen in haemolytic jaundice
D   there is reduced urinary bilirubin in hepatocellular jaundice
E   faecal stercobilinogen is increased in haemolytic jaundice.

XIX.23 **In familial periodic paralysis:**
A   attacks frequently occur during sleep
B   serum potassium is increased during attacks
C   high carbohydrate diet can precipitate an attack
D   attacks may be induced by infusion of glucose
E   patients are sensitive to depolarising neuromuscular blocking drugs.

XIX.24   Pharmacological effects of nicotine include:

A   hypotension
B   vasodilation
C   release of antidiuretic hormone
D   suppression of transmission through autonomic ganglia
E   respiratory stimulation.

XIX.25   The following are true of acute renal failure:

A   severe hypovolaemia is a cause
B   it can be diagnosed by a urinary specific gravity of 1010
C   frusemide 1–2 g intravenously can be given in the early stages
D   potassium supplements are needed
E   intravenous pyelography is useless.

XIX.26   The following are factors in the development of a lung abscess:

A   pharyngeal pouch
B   staphylococcal pneumonia
C   septicaemia
D   bronchopleural fistula
E   pulmonary embolism.

XIX.27   Common associations with primary bronchogenic carcinoma include:

A   finger clubbing
B   peripheral neuropathy
C   coin shadow on chest radiograph
D   palmar erythema
E   Horner's syndrome.

XIX.28   The following are true of ascites:

A   less than about 500 ml of fluid cannot be diagnosed clinically
B   it is most commonly caused by congestive cardiac failure
C   it is a poor prognostic sign in cirrhosis
D   it can be treated initially with diuretics
E   therapeutic paracentesis is contraindicated in malignant ascites.

XIX.29 **Oesophageal varices occur in:**
   A   achalasia of the cardia
   B   carcinoma of the oesophagus
   C   hepatic cirrhosis
   D   portal venous thrombosis
   E   chronic pancreatitis.

XIX.30 **The following factors delay union after fracture of a long bone:**
   A   malnutrition
   B   a fracture in a child of less than 9 months
   C   the site of the fracture
   D   pathological fracture
   E   a fracture in an adult of more than 60 years.

Paper XIX Answers

XIX.1 TFFTF

Temporary pacemakers are used less now than they were in the early 1980s.

A,D Episodes of heart block and transient unconsciousness of cardiac origin require treatment whether or not surgery is planned.

C This combination used to be an indication for temporary pacing during anaesthesia. It is not now an indication provided the patient is asymptomatic.

E Over-ride pacemakers are sometimes used for supraventricular tachyarrhythmias (but need for an anaesthetic is not an indication). The same applies to implanted defibrillators (which are not pacemakers).

XIX.2 TTFFT

C Esmolol is a short-acting drug that should be given by infusion for lengthy cases.

D A spinal anaesthetic would reduce the blood pressure, but is not a sensible approach when you consider the site of operation.

XIX.3 TTTTF

A,C Nitrous oxide diffuses into closed body compartments and worsens these serious conditions.

B Many anaesthetists switch on nitrous oxide without thinking. Bowel distension is a condition in which you should think.

D If a tympanic graft is overlaid on the eardrum, nitrous oxide will lift it off its bed. Most surgeons use an underlaid graft and here nitrous oxide may hold the graft in place. The answer, however, is 'true' as *there are occasions* when nitrous should not be used (see Q X.2).

E Prolonged exposure to nitrous oxide affects B_{12} metabolism, but that does not make this branch 'true'.

XIX.4   TFFFT

This is another clinical scenario: cover up the branches and work out what might be going on before looking at them.

A   Pulmonary collapse explains the findings. The hypercapnia may be partly due to opioid, but you are given no information about that.

B,D   Blood loss or over-transfusion will not cause the hypercapnia.

C   The slightly increased bicarbonate of 28 mmol/l excludes metabolic acidosis.

E   Hypercapnia is hypoventilation. (This is not inevitable: there may be greatly increased carbon dioxide production, but there is no reason for that here.)

XIX.5   TTTFT

D   Polycythaemic patients are not more susceptible than normal to Gram-negative septicaemia.

XIX.6   TTFFT

C,D   An infraclavicular approach has been described, but is not a *common* approach.

XIX.7   FTTTT

A   Sickle cell disease is not a contraindication to epidural anaesthesia.

E   This is a good topic for debate in a viva; different anaesthetists will have different opinions.

XIX.8   TFTFT

B   Steep head-down positions can cause unexpectedly high blocks.

C   This technique can lessen the decrease in pressure, but the safety of spinal catheters is uncertain at the time of writing.

D   Adrenaline can cause uterine artery vasoconstriction.

XIX.9   FFFTF

    A   Cryoanalgesia (freezing of the nerves) is used in pain relief clinics, but has gone out of fashion for treating acute pain because it can cause long-term dysaesthesia.

    B   Intercostal blocks would have to be bilateral and prolonged.

    C   Chlorocresol, a preservative used in drug ampoules, is neurolytic and can cause permanent neurological damage.

    E   Oral therapy is unsuitable after gastrointestinal surgery.

XIX.10   FTFTT

    A   Etomidate is the least likely of the induction agents to release histamine or cause allergic-type reactions.

    C   There is no evidence that etomidate is diabetogenic.

XIX.11   FTTFF

    A   Nitric oxide has a short half-life both in the environment and in the body.

    D   Nitric oxide is itself toxic.

    E   Nitric oxide relaxes all vascular smooth muscle. When inhaled, it affects only the pulmonary circulation because of rapid inactivation by haemoglobin.

XIX.12   TTTFF

There are many ways of giving an anaesthetic. The question asks whether the methods suggested are *reasonable*, not whether they are your choice.

    C   There is no reason to use nitrous oxide; but nor is there any special reason to avoid it.

    D   The peanut is likely to fragment during removal. Ventilation risks blowing fragments distally.

    E   Peanuts produce lytic enzymes which cause local oedema. Lavage spreads the enzymes further.

XIX.13   TTFTF

    B,C   The bicipital aponeurosis lies between the median cubital vein and the brachial artery.

    E   The brachial artery divides just distal to the elbow joint.

XIX.14 FTFFT

A   The median nerve is at risk from injections in the antecubital fossa, but not from positioning.

B   The saphenous is at risk from ankle straps at the medial malleolus.

C,D Neither the facial nor the trigeminal nerve is at risk.

E   The lateral popliteal is at risk at the neck of the fibula.

XIX.15 FTFTF

A   The length of the bevel has no effect on possible direct nerve damage.

C   The skin over the ischial tuberosity is innervated by the posterior primary rami.

D   The hamstrings will be affected as well.

XIX.16 TTTTF

B   Water is excreted because of the osmotic diuretic effect of the glucose.

D   Polyuric renal failure will cause hypernatraemia.

E   *Sweat* sodium, not serum sodium, is increased in cystic fibrosis.

XIX.17 TFTTT

An A–P film will be a portable X-ray rather than the usual departmental film.

B   A *pericardial*, but not a pleural, effusion will increase heart size.

D   Complete heart block will increase ventricular size because of increased filling time.

E   Heart size can be assessed accurately only on a P–A film.

XIX.18 TTFTF

C   In coarctation, a *late* systolic murmur extends into the second heart sound.

E   There is a pansystolic murmur in mitral regurgitation.

XIX.19   FTTFT

The 'a' wave reflects venous distension caused by right atrial contraction and is therefore absent if there is atrial flutter or fibrillation (**A,D**). They occur in ventricular tachycardia (**C**). Some, when the tricuspid valve is closed, are exaggerated, but generally they are not easy to see. Any obstruction to right ventricular emptying (**E**) exaggerates them.

XIX.20   TTFTF

C   Stridor is caused by thyroid *enlargement,* not hyperthyroidism.

E   A positive Chvostek's sign is a sign of low serum ionised calcium and may be found in hypoparathyroidism.

XIX.21   FTTFF

A   Anaemia is not an indication for urgent surgery in ulcerative colitis.

D   Steroids are a mainstay of medical treatment in acute flareups of ulcerative colitis.

E   Severe dehydration must be treated urgently before anaesthesia and surgery are safe.

XIX.22   TFFFT

MCQs on jaundice are common.

B   Urinary urobilinogen is normal or increased in hepatocellular jaundice unless there is obstruction.

C   Urinary urobilinogen is increased in haemolytic jaundice.

D   There is normal or increased urinary bilirubin in hepatocellular jaundice.

XIX.23   TFTTF

Familial periodic paralysis is a rare inherited condition that anaesthetists are unlikely to see but should be aware of.

B   During attacks serum potassium is normal or decreased.

E   There is a normal response to suxamethonium.

XIX.24   FFTTT

Nicotine is not a medicinal drug, but is of historical and theoretical importance in the pharmacology of the autonomic nervous system. Unfortunately, receptor physiology has become complex: once there was only one nicotinic and one muscarinic receptor, now new subtypes appear at disheartening intervals.

A,B   Nicotine causes cutaneous vasoconstriction, tachycardia and hypertension.

D   Transient stimulation of ganglia is followed by depression.

XIX.25   TFTFF

B   The urinary specific gravity may be 1010, but this value is not diagnostic of renal failure. A persistent SG of 1010 is more suggestive. There may be no urine at all.

C   It is uncertain whether frusemide affects the development of acute renal failure. Many use it.

D   Renal failure often causes *hyper*kalaemia.

E   Intravenous pyelography may show a nephrogram and can be helpful in diagnosis.

XIX.26   TTTTF

A   Aspiration is likely when there is a pharyngeal pouch.

C   Septic emboli can lodge in the lungs.

E   Pulmonary embolus is not a cause of lung abscess unless associated with sepsis.

XIX.27   TFFFF

Finger clubbing (**A**) is the only one of these that is a *common* association. All the others occur, but are unusual (see Q. XVII.26).

C   A round shadow is more likely to be a secondary.

XIX.28   TTFTF

C   Patients with stable cirrhosis can have ascites for years.

B,D   Diuretics are indicated when the ascites is caused by congestive cardiac failure. They can be used in patients with cirrhosis.

E   There is a risk of seeding when a malignant ascites is tapped, but relief of a patient's discomfort can outweigh the risk.

XIX.29   FFTTF

    A,B   Achalasia of the cardia is not associated with portal hypertension and varices.

    C,E   There is an indirect association (but not enough to give the answer as 'true') between chronic pancreatitis and varices, because chronic pancreatitis can be caused by alcoholism and cirrhosis.

XIX.30   TFTTF

    B,E   Young children heal quickly; once adult, age has little effect on union.

Paper XX   Questions

XX.1 **Likely complications of chair dental anaesthesia in the supine position include:**
A   regurgitation
B   postural hypotension
C   aspiration
D   cardiac arrhythmias
E   hypoglycaemia.

XX.2 **Vaporisers suitable for use in a drawover mode include:**
A   Tec mark 4
B   Oxford Miniature Vaporizer (OMV)
C   EMO
D   Goldman
E   Copper kettle.

XX.3 **The following are correct descriptions of the eye signs of anaesthesia:**
A   the eyelash reflex disappears in stage 2
B   the corneal reflex is absent throughout stage 3
C   eye movements are lost by plane 2 of stage 3
D   the pupillary light reflex is abolished in plane 3 of stage 3
E   mydriasis in stage 4 is caused by oculomotor paralysis.

XX.4 **Inherited diseases influencing elective general anaesthesia include:**
A   porphyria
B   malignant hyperpyrexia
C   atypical pseudocholinesterase
D   acromegaly
E   glucose-6-phosphate dehydrogenase deficiency.

XX.5 **A previously fit adult is hit by a car and is admitted with a compound fracture of the tibia but no other obvious injury. Despite good general condition, the patient fails to regain full consciousness, remaining drowsy and confused after correction of the fracture under uncomplicated general anaesthesia. Serious consideration should now be given to:**
A   subdural haematoma
B   cerebral fat embolism
C   bilateral pneumothorax
D   hypovolaemia requiring blood replacement
E   massive pulmonary embolism.

XX.6   When giving an anaesthetic for MRI scanning (magnetic resonance imaging):

A   a disposable plastic catheter mount must be used
B   cardiac pacemakers may malfunction
C   the anaesthetic machine must be fixed to the floor
D   a stethoscope should not be worn around the neck
E   ketamine sedation is contraindicated.

XX.7   In the Apgar scoring system of neonatal asphyxia:

A   a weak cry or hypoventilation scores 1
B   blue hands or feet scores 1
C   absent reflex responses scores 0
D   a heart rate above 80 scores 2
E   a single assessment at 1 min distinguishes primary from terminal apnoea.

XX.8   The following cause respiratory problems in the neonate:

A   choanal atresia
B   Pierre Robin syndrome
C   laryngomalacia
D   Treacher–Collins syndrome
E   cleft lip and palate.

XX.9   Patients with ankylosing spondylitis present for operation with the following recognised problems:

A   limited jaw gape
B   subluxation of the atlanto-axial joint
C   increased likelihood of anaphylactoid reactions
D   aortic regurgitation
E   peripheral vascular disease.

XX.10   A patient taking a monoamine oxidase inhibitor presents for elective hysterectomy. Anaesthetic management should include:

A   the avoidance of morphine premedication
B   rapid sequence induction of anaesthesia
C   subcutaneous heparin
D   preoperative beta-adrenergic blockade
E   cautious initial titration of pethidine as the opioid of choice.

XX.11 During one-lung anaesthesia:
A perfusion to the dependent lung increases
B ventilation to the dependent lung decreases
C ventilation/perfusion mismatching decreases when the diseased lung is collapsed
D anatomical dead space is reduced
E pulmonary vascular resistance is reduced.

XX.12 The following are true of the cervical plexus:
A it is formed from the anterior rami of all the cervical nerves
B there are in general three groups of branches of each ramus
C the largest contribution to the phrenic nerve is from C4
D the great auricular nerve has auricular, facial and mastoid branches
E C1 has only motor fibres.

XX.13 The following are true of the diaphragm:
A its development includes a muscular contribution from the cervical region
B there is somatic sensory innervation from the lower thoracic segments
C the arcuate ligaments insert into psoas major and quadratus lumborum
D the central tendon is smooth muscle
E its arterial supply is directly from the aorta.

XX.14 The mandibular division of the trigeminal nerve:
A subserves sensation from the posterior third of the tongue
B subserves cutaneous sensation approximately anterior to a line from the angle of the jaw through the external auditory meatus to the vertex
C is the only division of the trigeminal nerve with a true motor component
D carries salivary secretomotor fibres
E is the origin of the lingual nerve and inferior dental nerve.

XX.15 The following are true of the blood supply of the arm:
A the radial artery is usually larger than the ulnar artery
B the radial artery is usually palpated lateral to the tendon of flexor carpi ulnaris
C the radial artery helps form the deep palmar arch
D the ulnar artery crosses the flexor retinaculum
E the ulnar nerve lies medial to the ulnar artery at the wrist.

XX.16 The following statements are true of these haemodynamic measurements:

    A   normal left ventricular pressure is 120/4 mmHg

    B   the normal left-ventricular end-diastolic volume is 130 ml

    C   a pulmonary artery pressure of 25/10 mmHg is normal

    D   the normal left atrial pressure is 2–4 cm water

    E   capillary pressure at the start of a capillary is midway between arterial and venous pressures.

XX.17 Causes of pulmonary hypertension include:

    A   atrio-septal defect (ASD)

    B   chronic bronchitis

    C   pulmonary embolism

    D   sodium nitroprusside infusion

    E   high altitude.

XX.18 Clinical methods for detection of venous thrombosis include:

    A   venography

    B   Doppler ultrasound

    C   the use of radioactively labelled albumin

    D   impedance plethysmography

    E   labelled fibrinogen uptake.

XX.19 A 37-year-old diabetic taking a mixture of soluble and Lente insulin twice daily presents for major abdominal surgery. The following would be suitable perioperative regimens to keep his diabetes satisfactorily under control:

    A   a 10% dextrose infusion containing soluble insulin and potassium

    B   a depot injection of an ultra-long-acting insulin

    C   continue his normal injections and start intravenous feeding

    D   withhold insulin unless his blood sugar rises above 7 mmol/l

    E   soluble insulin on a timed sliding scale.

XX.20 A 17-year-old boy is admitted to hospital comatose. He is flushed, pyrexial and shows signs of cerebral irritability. The following are true:

    A   his trachea should be intubated if he has no gag reflex

    B   a lumbar puncture is indicated

    C   the blood glucose should be measured

    D   a radiograph of the skull should be obtained

    E   the signs are consistent with aspirin poisoning.

XX.21 **Likely causes of dysphagia lasting for some weeks include:**
A Plummer–Vinson syndrome
B pharyngeal pouch
C pseudobulbar palsy
D bronchogenic carcinoma
E oesophageal foreign body.

XX.22 **Vitamin K is useful in bleeding caused by:**
A haemophilia
B scurvy
C heparin overdosage
D oral anticoagulant overdosage
E factor XII deficiency.

XX.23 **A headache is unlikely to be of organic origin if:**
A it is aggravated by straining at stool
B the presentation is of mental depression
C it is unremitting and not localised
D it is worse in the morning
E a CT scan is normal.

XX.24 **Dextran solutions cause:**
A decreased coagulability
B antigenic reactions
C difficulties with cross-matching of blood type
D damage to renal tubules
E rouleaux formation of red blood cells.

XX.25 **In chronic respiratory acidosis with renal compensation:**
A arterial pH is decreased
B $PaCO_2$ is increased
C base excess is increased
D standard bicarbonate is decreased
E blood CO_2 content is decreased.

XX.26   A reduced FEV$_1$/FVC ratio occurs:

A   in restrictive lung disease
B   in obstructive lung disease
C   when the static compliance is decreased
D   in children
E   in fibrosing alveolitis.

XX.27   Factors in the development of acute pancreatitis include:

A   haemochromatosis
B   previous gastrectomy
C   uraemia
D   halothane anaesthesia
E   hypocalcaemia.

XX.28   The characteristic pain of duodenal ulcer is:

A   episodic
B   associated with vomiting
C   worse at night
D   exacerbated by smoking
E   associated with weight loss.

XX.29   The following are true of carcinoma of the rectum:

A   blood-borne metastasis occurs late
B   the adrenal gland is a site of secondaries
C   bleeding is a common early symptom
D   pain is an early symptom
E   ascites indicates hepatic secondaries.

XX.30   Postoperative retention of urine:

A   is common after haemorrhoidectomy
B   is less likely with effective opioid epidural analgesia
C   is more likely with spinal anaesthesia
D   should be treated initially with a single dose of frusemide
E   is frequently painless.

Paper XX   Answers

XX.1   TFTTF
B   Postural hypotension is not a complication of the supine position.
D   Arrhythmias are most likely if the inhalational agent is halothane.
E   Unless a patient is diabetic, hypoglycaemia will not occur.

XX.2   FTTTF
A,E   Drawover vaporisers must be of low resistance. The Tec series and the Copper kettle (still used for calibration) are not and are suitable only for plenum use.
C,D   The EMO (Epstein–Macintosh–Oxford) and the Goldman are now rarely used in developed countries.

XX.3   TFTTF
There are other questions in this book relating to the classical Guedel signs of anaesthesia (see Q III.4). They are not directly relevant to modern 'balanced' anaesthesia, but are of great historical importance and the principles are worth learning.
A   The lash reflex disappears in plane 2 of stage 3.
E   Mydriasis in stage 4 is due to deep CNS depression (and, as was practised then, hypoxia). Oculomotor paralysis occurs in plane 2 of stage 3.

XX.4   TTTFT
Questions commonly ask about the methods of inheritance of these conditions. While the inheritance is interesting (and as a career anaesthetist you should be interested to know), it is more important to know in what way these conditions put patients at risk and how any risk can be reduced or avoided.
D   Acromegaly is not inherited.

XX.5   TTFFF
C–E   The key phrase is 'despite good general condition'. This rules out pneumothorax, hypovolaemia and pulmonary embolus.

XX.6   TTTTF

A   Catheter mounts must be plastic to avoid interfering with the image. Most anaesthetists believe that the airway should be secured by endotracheal tube if an anaesthetic is to be given: access to the head is poor on most current machines.

C   The anaesthetic machine must be a regulation distance outside the magnetic field.

D   The stethoscope could be attracted (rapidly) into the magnetic field.

E   Ketamine can be used provided that the airway can be controlled.

XX.7   TTTFF

D   A heart rate above 100 scores 2.

E   A single assessment cannot distinguish primary from terminal apnoea. Primary apnoea at 1 min can recover spontaneously, while terminal apnoea will require treatment.

XX.8   TTTTF

E   Cleft lip and palate cause problems with feeding, but not usually with respiration.

XX.9   TTFTF

C   Ankylosing spondylitis is an autoimmune disease but anaphylactoid reactions are no more or less likely than in anyone else.

D   Patients who have had ankylosing spondylitis for many years sometimes develop an aortitis and damage to the aortic valve.

E   There is no association between ankylosing spondylitis and peripheral vascular disease.

XX.10 TFFFF

A,E   The initial use of any opioid should be very cautious with careful monitoring of blood pressure. Pethidine is contraindicated.

B   There is no special indication for rapid sequence induction.

C,D   These are not always indicated. Some gynaecologists give subcutaneous heparin to all patients undergoing hysterectomies.

XX.11   TFTTF

B   Ventilation must at least remain the same, but usually increases, especially if the patient is being artificially ventilated.

E   The circulation of the two lungs is in parallel. When one lung is taken out of circuit, the overall resistance increases.

XX.12   FFTTT

A   The cervical plexus is formed from the anterior rami of C1–4.

B   The *four* general groups of branches are the communicating, superficial, deep and phrenic. They are 'general' because not all rami divide to give all four groups.

XX.13   TTTFF

A   The motor supply is (mostly) from the phrenic nerve (C3–5).

D   The central tendon is fibrous, but the muscle of the diaphragm is all striated muscle.

E   The arterial supply of the diaphragm is small print. The supply is complex: there are musculophrenic, superior and inferior phrenic arteries, and further supply from the intercostal arteries.

XX.14   FTTTT

A   The trigeminal nerve subserves sensation from the *anterior two-thirds* of the tongue.

D   The secretomotor fibres originate in the facial nerve and travel via the chorda tympani.

XX.15   FTTTT

A   The radial artery is the more direct continuation of the brachial, and is the choice for cannulation; but the ulnar artery is usually the larger.

C   The radial artery anastomoses with the deep branch of the ulnar artery to form the deep palmar arch.

XX.16   TTTFF

  A   An unfamiliar measurement, although left ventricular catheters are sometimes used after cardiac surgery.

  D   The normal left atrial pressure is 8–10 cm water.

  E   Most of the pressure drop occurs in the arterioles. Start-capillary pressure (about 25 mmHg) is much less than midway between arterial and venous pressures.

XX.17   TTTFT

  A   The hyperdynamic circulation of an ASD causes pulmonary hypertension.

  B,E   Vasoconstriction secondary to hypoxia causes pulmonary hypertension in chronic bronchitis and at high altitude.

  D   Sodium nitroprusside decreases both pulmonary and systemic blood pressures.

XX.18   TTFFT

  C,D   Radioactively labelled albumin and impedance plethysmography have both been used, but are not clinical methods.

XX.19   TFFFT

  The two previous questions on diabetes (Q V.2, IX.2) have been about non-insulin-dependent diabetes.

  A,E   Both are effective but continuous infusion is in favour at the moment. Dextrose can be given with the infusion ('Alberti regimen') or separately.

  B   There is no place for long-acting insulins in the perioperative period.

  C   Feeding, if required, will increase insulin requirements and should be used in conjunction with an insulin infusion.

  D   Insulin should not be withheld from insulin-dependent diabetics.

XX.20   TTTFF

  B   Lumbar puncture may show meningitis or encephalitis. A lumbar puncture is easy to do and a sensible precaution in any undiagnosed coma (provided there are not obvious signs of raised intracranial pressure).

  D   A skull X-ray is not necessary unless there is a history of head injury.

  E   Coma after aspirin overdose is rare except in children. It can cause convulsions, but why should he be flushed and pyrexial? But don't forget that some recreational drugs may produce this picture.

XX.21   TTTTF
- **A**   In Plummer–Vinson syndrome there is an oesophageal web.
- **D**   Bronchogenic carcinoma causes dysphagia by compression.
- **E**   A foreign body is unlikely to cause dysphagia that lasts more than a few days before diagnosis.

XX.22   FFFTF
- **A**   Factor VIII is not dependent on vitamin K.
- **B**   Scurvy is vitamin C deficiency, in which there is capillary fragility.
- **C**   Heparin does not affect prothrombin.
- **E**   Factor XII is not prothrombin-dependent.

XX.23   FFTFF
- **A,D**   A headache made worse by straining and worse in the morning are both signs of increased intracranial pressure.
- **B**   Depressed patients get headaches, but frontal lobe tumours in particular present with mental change.
- **C**   The classical psychoneurotic headache: *but* a dangerous diagnosis to make hastily.
- **E**   There are many organic causes in which a CT scan would be entirely normal.

XX.24   TTTTF
Dextrans (long-chain starch solutions) have been largely replaced by denatured collagens – because of the problems asked in this question.
- **A**   Dextrans reduce platelet aggregation (which is why Dextran 70 is still used during vascular surgery), destabilise fibrin and activate plasmin.
- **B**   The incidence of allergic-type reactions is higher with Dextrans than with collagens.
- **D**   Dextran 40 caused occasional acute renal failure.
- **E**   Dextrans reduce rouleaux formation; rouleaux form in *dextrose* solutions.

XX.25   TTTFF
- **A**   Compensation is never complete, so the pH will still be lower than normal.
- **D**   Renal compensation retains bicarbonate.
- **E**   Blood CO_2 content will be increased.

XX.26   FTFFF

A,E   The absolute values of FEV_1 and FVC are reduced in restrictive disease, but the ratio is normal.

C   Increases in airways *resistance* reduce the ratio.

XX.27   TTTFF

D   There is no association of halothane and pancreatitis.

E   Long-standing *hyper*calcaemia is a cause of acute pancreatitis. *Hypo*calcaemia *occurs in* the disease.

XX.28   TFTTF

A   The pain typically occurs for a few days and is then followed by weeks free of pain.

B,E   Vomiting and weight loss are characteristic of *gastric* ulcer.

XX.29   TTTFF

B   Liver and lungs are the commonest site of secondaries from rectal carcinoma. Secondaries do occur in the adrenals.

C,D   Bleeding is the *commonest* early symptom. Pain usually occurs late.

E   Ascites may be because of liver secondaries, but peritoneal seedlings are the more likely cause.

XX.30   TFTFF

B,C   Both spinal and epidural analgesia increase the risk of urinary retention.

D   Frusemide is given too often postoperatively. When patients are oliguric because they have not been given enough fluid, frusemide is bad medicine. It is verging on the negligent to give frusemide to a patient *known or suspected to be* in retention.

E   Patients are commonly in pain and very restless. There is the danger that effective regional analgesia will block the pain of retention.

Index

Questions are listed under broad headings only. There is some overlap between categories; no question is listed more than once. Roman numerals indicate the number of the paper, and the arabic number that follows is the number of the question on the paper.

Anaesthesia